The Complete Gastric Sleeve Bariatric Air Fryer Cookbook For Beginners

2000+ Days of Flavorful, Simple and Fast Recipes for Rapid Weight Loss and Lasting Health Post-Surgery | 90-Day Meal Plan.

By Olivia Serrano

Table Of Contents

CHAPTER 1: INTRODUCTION 9

Understanding Gastric Sleeve Surgery 9

The Role of Diet Post-Surgery 11

Why the Air Fryer is a Game-Changer 13

CHAPTER 2: GASTRIC SLEEVE AND NUTRITION 15

Essentials of Post-Surgery Nutrition 15

Foods to Embrace and Foods to Avoid 17

Meeting Nutritional Needs: Protein, Vitamins, and More 19

The Importance of Portion Control 22

CHAPTER 3: MASTERING YOUR AIR FRYER 24

The Benefits of Air Frying Post-Surgery 24

Getting to Know Your Air Fryer 27

Tips and Tricks for Perfect Air Frying Every Time 29

CHAPTER 4: RECIPES 31

Phase 1: Liquid Diet Recipes - Nourishing Broths 31
    Golden Turmeric Bone Broth 31
    Healing Ginger Chicken Broth 31
    Soothing Lemongrass Beef Broth 32
    Mint and Lamb Healing Broth 32
    Citrus-Infused Fish Broth 34
    Spicy Tomato and Bone Broth 34
    Herbal Turkey Broth 35
    Asian-Style Pork Broth 35
    Rosemary and Veal Bone Broth 36
    Zingy Pepper and Chicken Broth 36
    Cilantro Lime Seafood Broth 37
    Earthy Mushroom and Garlic Broth 37
    Soothing Carrot and Ginger Broth 38
    Invigorating Peppermint and Lamb Broth 38

Ginger Infused Chicken Broth 39

Nutritious Smoothies and Juices 40

Antioxidant Berry Blast Smoothie 40

Green Detox Juice 40

Tropical Mango Smoothie 40

Soothing Almond Milk and Vanilla Shake 41

Red Beet and Berry Juice 41

Carrot and Ginger Zinger Juice 41

Creamy Avocado and Spinach Smoothie 42

Blueberry Oatmeal Breakfast Smoothie 42

Refreshing Cucumber and Lime Juice 42

Pineapple and Ginger Immune Booster 43

Protein-Packed Chocolate Almond Shake 43

Vibrant Veggie Green Juice 43

Golden Milk Turmeric Smoothie 44

Spiced Apple Cinnamon Juice 44

Strawberry Kiwi Hydration Smoothie 44

Phase 2: Pureed and Soft Foods - Pureed Vegetables 45

Roasted Carrot and Ginger Puree 45

Creamy Broccoli and Avocado Blend 45

Pumpkin and White Bean Mousse 46

Smooth Zucchini and Basil Blend 46

Velvety Beet and Yogurt Puree 47

Cauliflower and Chive Cream 47

Sweet Potato and Cinnamon Mash 48

Savory Lentil and Carrot Cream 48

Pea and Mint Puree 48

Roasted Red Pepper and Walnut Spread 49

Soft and Creamy Breakfast Options 49

Apple Cinnamon Oatmeal Puree 49

Berry Yogurt Bliss 50

Creamy Avocado and Banana Smoothie 50

Peaches and Cream Oatmeal 50

Silken Tofu and Berry Pudding 51

Mango Coconut Rice Pudding 51

Pumpkin Spice Smoothie 52

Almond Butter and Jelly Oatmeal 52

Cinnamon Apple Quinoa Porridge 53

Sweet Potato and Maple Mash 53

Gentle Snacks and Appetizers 54

Carrot and Coriander Soup 54

Creamy Avocado Dip 54

Mashed Pea and Mint Spread 55

Roasted Red Pepper Hummus 55

Baked Apple and Cinnamon Puree 56

Sweet Potato and Ginger Soup 56

Pumpkin and Nutmeg Mousse 57
Creamy Beet and Feta Dip 57
Zucchini and Basil Velouté 58
Cauliflower and Parmesan Cream 58

Phase 3: Transition to Solid Foods - Poultry and Meat 59
Herb-Infused Chicken Breast 59
Lemon Garlic Turkey Tenderloin 59
Spiced Ground Chicken Patties 60
Rosemary and Thyme Turkey Meatballs 60
Tender BBQ Chicken Thighs 61
Garlic Herb Roasted Turkey Breast 61
Balsamic Glazed Chicken Drumsticks 62
Simple Lemon Pepper Chicken Wings 62
Soy Glazed Turkey Meatloaf 63
Honey Mustard Chicken Tenders 63

Fish & Seafood 64
Lemon Herb Air-Fried Salmon 64
Garlic Butter Air-Fried Shrimp 64
Crispy Air-Fried Tilapia 65
Spiced Cod Air-Fryer Delight 65
Herbed Shrimp and Asparagus 66
Air-Fried Flounder with Lemon Pepper 66
Simple Air-Fried Scallops 67
Lime Cilantro Air-Fried Haddock 67
Tarragon Air-Fried Salmon Patties 68
Sweet and Sour Air-Fried Shrimp 68

Desserts & Sweets 69
Air-Fried Cinnamon Apples 69
Banana Nut Soft Bake 69
Air-Fried Peach Crumble 70
Soft Baked Pear with Honey 70
Vanilla and Berry Compote 71
Chocolate Avocado Pudding 71
Air-Fried Mango Slices 71
Cinnamon Ricotta Cream 72
Air-Fried Stuffed Apples 72
Soft Berry Sorbet 73

CHAPTER 5: SPECIAL DIETARY CONSIDERATIONS 74

Recipes for Lactose Intolerance 74
Phase 1 | Almond Milk and Berry Smoothie 74
Phase 2 | Creamy Pumpkin Soup 74
Phase 3 | Lactose-Free Chicken Parmesan 75
Phase 1 | Lactose-Free Protein Shake 75
Phase 2 | Mashed Cauliflower and Garlic 76

Phase 3 | Dairy-Free Beef Stroganoff 76
Phase 1 | Lactose-Free Berry Yogurt Smoothie 77
Phase 2 | Dairy-Free Avocado Cream Soup 77
Phase 3 | Lactose-Free Thai Curry Chicken 78
Phase 1 | Lactose-Free Creamy Carrot Ginger Juice 78

Gluten-Free and Low-Sugar Options 79
Phase 1 | Quinoa Breakfast Bowl 79
Phase 2 | Gluten-Free Veggie Omelette 79
Phase 3 | Low-Sugar Teriyaki Salmon 80
Phase 1 | Almond Butter Banana Smoothie 80
Phase 2 | Quinoa Stuffed Bell Peppers 81
Phase 3 | Low-Sugar Berry Parfait 81
Phase 1 | Gluten-Free Pancakes 82
Phase 2 | Gluten-Free Spinach and Feta Omelette 82
Phase 3 | Low-Sugar Grilled Pineapple 83
Phase 1 | Gluten-Free Banana Muffins 83

CHAPTER 6: 90-DAY MEAL PLANNER 84

10-Day Meal Plan: Phase 1 - Liquid Diet 84

10-Day Meal Plan: Phase 1 - Liquid Diet (Days 11-20) 85

10-Day Meal Plan: Phase 1 - Liquid Diet (Days 21-30) 86

10-Day Meal Plan: Phase 2 - Pureed and Soft Foods (Days 31-40) 87

10-Day Meal Plan: Phase 2 - Pureed and Soft Foods (Days 41-50) 88

10-Day Meal Plan: Phase 3 - Transition to Solid Foods (Days 51-60) 89

10-Day Meal Plan: Phase 3 - Transition to Solid Foods (Days 61-70) 90

10-Day Meal Plan: Phase 3 - Transition to Solid Foods (Days 71-80) 91

10-Day Meal Plan: Phase 3 - Transition to Solid Foods (Days 81-90) 92

CHAPTER 7: MAINTENANCE AND MOVING FORWARD 93

Staying on Track: The Art of Long-Term Success 93

Addressing Common Challenges: Navigating the Bumps in the Road 96

Celebrating Milestones and Successes: Acknowledging Your Achievements 100

CONCLUSION & YOUR NEXT STEPS: A JOURNEY BEYOND SURGERY 102

ACKNOWLEDGMENTS: GRATITUDE FOR SUPPORT AND INSPIRATION 104

Chapter 1: Introduction

Understanding Gastric Sleeve Surgery

Embarking on a journey through gastric sleeve surgery is not just a medical decision; it's a step towards a new chapter in life. This procedure, known medically as sleeve gastrectomy, has emerged as a beacon of hope for many grappling with weight-related challenges and its associated health risks. But what exactly is gastric sleeve surgery, and what does it entail for those who choose this path?

This surgery is more than a medical procedure; it's a commitment to a lifelong change. It involves the removal of a significant portion of the stomach, approximately 80%, leaving a banana-shaped "sleeve" that serves as the new stomach. This drastic reduction in stomach size naturally limits food intake, aiding in significant weight loss. But the impact of gastric sleeve surgery extends beyond physical transformation. It's a gateway to a renewed lifestyle, a promise of a healthier future.

The decision to undergo gastric sleeve surgery is often laden with a mixture of emotions - hope, anxiety, excitement, and concern. It's a journey that begins much before the surgery itself, often involving consultations with doctors, nutritionists, and even psychologists. Understanding the nuances of this surgery is pivotal, not just for the physical preparation but for mental readiness as well.

One might wonder, what leads an individual to choose gastric sleeve surgery? The reasons are manifold. For many, it's a decision fueled by the struggle with obesity and its accompanying health risks like diabetes, hypertension, and heart disease. For others, it's about enhancing quality of life, gaining mobility, and breaking free from the shackles of weight that have held them back. It's about reclaiming control over their health and, by extension, their lives.

The surgery itself is a marvel of modern medicine, typically performed laparoscopically. This minimally invasive approach involves small incisions and the use of a camera and instruments to remove part of the stomach. The benefits of a laparoscopic approach are significant - reduced pain, shorter hospital stay, and quicker recovery. However, it's essential to acknowledge that the surgery is not a quick fix. It's a tool, a powerful one indeed, but its effectiveness lies in how it's used in the grand tapestry of lifestyle changes.

Post-surgery, the real work begins. The newly shaped stomach necessitates a complete overhaul of eating habits. The first few weeks are marked by a liquid diet, gradually transitioning to pureed foods, and eventually, solids. This progression is crucial, allowing the body to adapt to its new anatomy. Portion control becomes a cornerstone of the post-surgery diet, with an emphasis on high-protein, low-carbohydrate foods.

The changes, however, are not confined to diet alone. Gastric sleeve surgery demands a holistic approach to health. Regular exercise, hydration, vitamin and mineral supplementation, and constant monitoring of nutritional intake become integral parts of daily life. But it's not just about adhering to a regimen; it's about embracing a new perspective on health and wellness.

The emotional and psychological aspects of life post-surgery are as significant as the physical ones. Many individuals experience a surge in confidence and self-esteem as they witness the transformation in their bodies. However, it's not uncommon to encounter emotional challenges. Adjusting to a new body image, coping with dietary restrictions, and dealing with the reactions of others can be overwhelming. Support groups, counseling, and open conversations with healthcare providers become vital in navigating these emotional waters.

The Role of Diet Post-Surgery

After the physical transformation initiated by gastric sleeve surgery, the role of diet emerges as the protagonist in this new chapter of life. The significance of dietary changes post-surgery cannot be overstated. It's a journey that involves relearning, rediscovery, and a deep commitment to nourishment.

The immediate aftermath of surgery ushers in a period of adjustment. The body, now adapting to a smaller stomach, requires a diet that is not only mindful of quantity but also of quality. This period is often characterized by a structured dietary plan, meticulously designed to aid healing and facilitate the body's adjustment to its new state.

Initially, the diet is liquid, gently nudging the body into acceptance of its new normal. This phase, though temporary, is critical. It's a time when hydration takes precedence, and nutrients are delivered in their simplest form. As the weeks progress, the dietary plan evolves, moving from pureed foods to soft solids, and eventually, to a more regular diet. Each stage is a stepping stone, a crucial part of the healing process.

The essence of the post-surgery diet lies in its composition. High-protein foods take center stage, providing the building blocks for healing and maintenance of muscle mass. Carbohydrates, particularly simple carbs, are significantly reduced, aligning with the body's decreased capacity to handle large quantities of food. Healthy fats are incorporated in moderation, offering essential fatty acids and aiding in the absorption of fat-soluble vitamins.

Portion control emerges as a key theme. With a smaller stomach, the quantity of food that can be comfortably consumed in one sitting is vastly reduced. This necessitates a shift in eating habits – smaller, more frequent meals replace the traditional three large meals a day. It's a change that requires mindfulness and discipline, retraining the mind to understand the new limits of the body.

But the role of diet extends beyond the physical aspects. It's also about forging a new relationship with food. For many, the journey to gastric sleeve surgery is intertwined with emotional eating, using food as a coping mechanism for stress, anxiety, or depression. Post-surgery, there's an opportunity to break free from these patterns, to learn to view food as nourishment rather than an emotional crutch.

This new relationship with food also involves exploring flavors and textures, discovering that healthy food can be both nourishing and enjoyable. It's about learning to savor each bite, to appreciate the aromas, the tastes, and the experience of eating. This is where the joy of cooking and the art of meal preparation come into play, transforming the necessity of eating into an enjoyable, life-affirming activity.

Nutritional education becomes an indispensable tool. Understanding the components of food, the role of different nutrients, and the importance of balanced meals is crucial. This knowledge empowers individuals to make informed choices, to build meals that are satisfying, nutritious, and in harmony with their new dietary needs.

Why the Air Fryer is a Game-Changer

So, what makes the air fryer an indispensable ally in this journey? The answer lies in its unique cooking method. The air fryer uses hot air to cook food, requiring little to no oil. This method not only reduces the calorie content of meals but also helps in avoiding the heavy, greasy feeling that can be particularly uncomfortable for those with a reduced stomach size. It's a way to enjoy the texture and taste of fried foods without the drawbacks associated with traditional frying methods.

The versatility of the air fryer is remarkable. It can be used to cook a wide range of foods – from vegetables and meats to even baked goods. This versatility is particularly valuable post-surgery, where dietary variety can be challenging due to the reduced stomach capacity and specific nutritional needs. The air fryer makes it possible to explore a wide array of recipes, ensuring that meals remain interesting and flavorful, a crucial factor in long-term dietary satisfaction and adherence.

Another advantage of the air fryer is its efficiency and convenience. In the busy lives of those adjusting to a new lifestyle post-surgery, time and ease of meal preparation are significant considerations. The air fryer heats up quickly and cooks food faster than traditional ovens. It's a time-saver, a feature that aligns perfectly with the needs of individuals looking for quick, healthy meal options.

Moreover, the air fryer is user-friendly and safe. With straightforward settings and a contained cooking environment, it reduces the risk of cooking-related accidents, a feature especially beneficial for those who might be new to cooking or have limited experience in the kitchen. Its ease of use encourages experimentation and confidence in meal preparation, empowering individuals to take an active role in their diet.

Clean-up is another aspect where the air fryer shines. Its parts are generally dishwasher-safe, making the post-meal clean-up a breeze. This ease of maintenance further adds to its appeal, especially for those who find cleaning a cumbersome task after a long day.

But perhaps the most significant contribution of the air fryer in the context of post-gastric sleeve surgery is its role in making healthy eating enjoyable. The texture of food matters, and the air fryer excels in providing that desirable crispness and flavor that can make healthy foods more appealing. It opens up a world where eating healthily doesn't mean compromising on taste or food enjoyment.

Chapter 2: Gastric Sleeve and Nutrition

Essentials of Post-Surgery Nutrition

Nutrition after gastric sleeve surgery isn't just a component of recovery; it's the foundation upon which a new lifestyle is built. This journey is less about restriction and more about transformation – a transformation that is both profound and deeply personal. Understanding the essentials of post-surgery nutrition is not just about following a set of guidelines; it's about embracing a new way of relating to food.

Post-surgery, the body undergoes significant changes, not just in its capacity to hold food but also in how it absorbs and processes nutrients. The reduced size of the stomach calls for a complete overhaul of eating habits. This isn't a temporary shift; it's a permanent change, a lifelong commitment to nourishing the body differently.

The first and foremost aspect of post-surgery nutrition is the emphasis on protein. Protein is the building block of the body – it aids in healing post-surgery, helps maintain muscle mass, and keeps you feeling full longer. The challenge, however, lies in consuming enough protein within the constraints of a smaller stomach. This requires thoughtful meal planning, ensuring that high-protein foods are prioritized. Foods like lean meats, eggs, low-fat dairy products, and legumes become staples in the diet. The goal is to include protein in every meal, making it the centerpiece around which other components are added.

However, the emphasis on protein doesn't diminish the importance of other nutrients. Carbohydrates are still a part of the diet but in a much-altered form.

Complex carbohydrates, found in foods like vegetables, whole grains, and fruits, should be chosen over simple carbs. These complex carbs are packed with fiber, aiding digestion, and providing essential nutrients without causing rapid spikes in blood sugar levels.

Fats are another crucial element, but the type of fat matters immensely. Post-gastric sleeve surgery, the focus should be on healthy fats – those found in avocados, nuts, seeds, and olive oil. These fats are not just sources of energy; they're vital for the absorption of fat-soluble vitamins and for maintaining healthy skin, hair, and organs.

Vitamins and minerals take on a new level of importance post-surgery. The body's ability to absorb certain nutrients is reduced, making supplementation a key aspect of post-surgery nutrition. Vitamins like B12, D, A, and minerals like iron and calcium often require supplementation. It's not just about popping pills; it's about understanding the body's new needs and addressing them proactively.

Hydration is another cornerstone of post-surgery nutrition. With a smaller stomach, the risk of dehydration increases. Drinking enough water throughout the day is crucial, but it's equally important to time it right – drinking before or after meals rather than during, to avoid filling up the stomach with fluids instead of nutrient-dense foods.

The transition to this new way of eating isn't just physical; it's deeply psychological. It requires breaking old habits, relearning hunger cues, and understanding satiety in a new light. It's about developing a mindful approach to eating – savoring each bite, eating slowly, and listening to the body's signals. This mindfulness extends to meal preparation as well – choosing ingredients thoughtfully, cooking in ways that preserve nutrients, and presenting food in a manner that delights the senses.

Foods to Embrace and Foods to Avoid

Navigating the post-gastric sleeve dietary landscape is akin to embarking on a culinary journey, one that requires a map to guide through the terrains of what to eat and what to avoid. This journey is not just about avoiding certain foods; it's about discovering a whole new spectrum of ingredients that can enrich your life.

Foods to Embrace

1. **Lean Proteins:** The stars of your post-surgery diet, lean proteins are not just vital for healing but also for maintaining muscle mass and overall health. Think of grilled chicken, fish, turkey, tofu, and eggs. These foods provide the necessary nutrients without the burden of excess fat.

2. **Vegetables and Fruits:** These natural treasures are sources of essential vitamins, minerals, and fiber. However, their intake must be balanced, especially in the early stages post-surgery. Focus on non-starchy vegetables like leafy greens, broccoli, and bell peppers. Fruits should be consumed in moderation due to their sugar content; opt for low-glycemic options like berries, apples, and pears.

3. **Whole Grains:** While your intake of carbohydrates needs to be moderated, whole grains are a beneficial part of your diet. Foods like quinoa, barley, and whole wheat provide fiber and other nutrients, aiding digestion and adding a sense of fullness.

4. **Healthy Fats:** Incorporating healthy fats is key. Avocados, nuts, seeds, and olive oil are excellent choices, providing essential fatty acids and aiding in the absorption of vitamins.

5. **Low-fat Dairy Products:** These are important for their calcium content. Opt for low-fat or fat-free options to get the benefit of calcium without the added fats.

Foods to Avoid

1. **High-fat Foods:** Post-surgery, your body may have difficulty processing high-fat foods. Foods like fried foods, full-fat dairy products, and fatty cuts of meat should be avoided.
2. **Sugary Foods and Drinks:** Excess sugar can lead to "dumping syndrome," causing discomfort, nausea, and dizziness. Avoid sugary snacks, sodas, and even some fruits with high sugar content.
3. **Highly Processed Foods:** These are often high in calories, fats, and sugars but low in nutritional value. They can disrupt your weight loss progress and overall health goals.
4. **Alcohol:** Alcohol can be harsh on your new stomach and also high in empty calories. It's best to avoid it, especially in the early stages post-surgery.
5. **Carbonated Beverages:** These can cause bloating and discomfort, as well as stretch your stomach over time. Stick to water, herbal teas, and other non-carbonated beverages.

Adopting this new approach to eating is not just about following a list of dos and don'ts; it's about making choices that align with your health goals. It's about understanding that every food you consume has a direct impact on your well-being.

Meeting Nutritional Needs: Protein, Vitamins, and More

Protein is the cornerstone of your post-surgery diet. Its importance cannot be overstated – it's crucial for healing, maintaining muscle mass, and ensuring overall health. But how do you ensure adequate protein intake when your stomach's capacity is significantly reduced?

The key is to incorporate protein-rich foods in every meal. Options like lean meats, poultry, fish, eggs, low-fat dairy products, and plant-based proteins like beans and lentils should be staples in your diet. For some, protein supplements may be necessary, especially in the early stages post-surgery when food intake is limited. These supplements should be carefully chosen – low in sugar and high in protein, ideally whey or plant-based proteins.

Vitamins and Minerals: The Unsung Heroes

Vitamins and minerals are the unsung heroes of your post-surgery nutrition. Given the reduced capacity to consume large quantities of food and potential changes in absorption, deficiencies in vitamins and minerals are a real concern.

Key vitamins and minerals to focus on include:

- Vitamin B12: Essential for nerve function and the production of DNA and red blood cells.
- Iron: Crucial for the formation of red blood cells and the prevention of anemia.
- Calcium and Vitamin D: Vital for bone health, especially important as rapid weight loss can affect bone density.

- Multivitamins: A broad-spectrum multivitamin can help cover the bases for various other vitamins and minerals.

Supplementation of these nutrients is often necessary. However, it's important to work with a healthcare provider to determine the right supplements and dosages, as individual needs can vary greatly.

Hydration: The Essence of Life

Hydration takes on a new level of importance after gastric sleeve surgery. The body's signals for thirst and hunger can often be confused, and with the reduced stomach size, there's less room for both food and liquids.

Aim for at least 64 ounces of fluid per day, primarily in the form of water. However, this intake should be spread out throughout the day. Drinking too much liquid at once can lead to discomfort and even stretching of the stomach. Avoid drinking fluids 30 minutes before and after meals to ensure that you can eat enough nutrient-rich foods.

Fiber: The Balancing Act

Fiber plays a critical role in digestion and regularity, something that can be a concern post-surgery. However, the introduction of fiber must be gradual to avoid gastrointestinal discomfort. Focus on incorporating non-starchy vegetables and eventually small portions of fruits and whole grains. This gradual introduction will help your digestive system adjust without causing discomfort.

Listening to Your Body

Post-surgery, your body's signals can be a reliable guide. Pay attention to signs of deficiency, which can include fatigue, hair loss, dry skin, and mood changes. Regular blood work is essential to monitor nutrient levels and make adjustments as needed.

Remember, meeting your nutritional needs post-gastric sleeve surgery is a dynamic process. It requires attention, adjustment, and sometimes, patience.

The Importance of Portion Control

Portion control is essential for ensuring that your reduced stomach capacity is not overwhelmed, while also providing your body with the nutrients it needs to heal and thrive.

Redefining Fullness

After gastric sleeve surgery, the concept of fullness takes on a new meaning. Your stomach, now significantly smaller, signals fullness much sooner than before. The challenge lies in learning to understand and respect these new signals. It's a process that requires mindfulness and patience. Overeating can lead not only to discomfort but also to stretching of the stomach over time, potentially undermining the benefits of the surgery.

Measuring and Planning: Keys to Success

Measuring food portions becomes an integral part of your daily routine. Using measuring cups, spoons, and food scales can help you accurately gauge portion sizes. But portion control isn't just about measuring; it's also about planning. Planning your meals ahead of time ensures that you have the right amount of food, reducing the temptation to overeat.

In the initial weeks and months post-surgery, your healthcare team will provide specific guidelines on portion sizes. Typically, meals will start small - sometimes as little as a few tablespoons - and gradually increase as your stomach heals. It's crucial to adhere to these guidelines, as they are designed to maximize healing and minimize discomfort.

The Role of Frequency in Eating

With the necessity of smaller portions comes the need to eat more frequently. Instead of three large meals, you'll likely find yourself eating five to six smaller meals throughout the day. This approach ensures a steady intake of nutrients and helps maintain energy levels. It also helps in managing hunger, as waiting too long between meals can lead to overeating.

Visual Cues and Mindful Eating

Visual cues can be incredibly helpful in maintaining portion control. Smaller plates, bowls, and utensils can make your portions appear larger, providing psychological satisfaction. Mindful eating practices, such as eating slowly, chewing thoroughly, and savoring each bite, can also aid in recognizing fullness cues.

The Psychological Aspect of Portion Control

Portion control is as much a psychological challenge as it is a physical one. It requires breaking long-held habits and beliefs about meal sizes. Many people equate larger portions with more satisfaction, a notion that must be reevaluated. Learning to find satisfaction in smaller quantities is a gradual process, one that involves retraining both the mind and the body.

The Long-Term Perspective

Portion control is not a temporary phase; it's a lifelong commitment. As you progress further from your surgery date, maintaining portion control becomes critical for sustaining weight loss and promoting overall health. It's about creating and maintaining a balanced relationship with food, one where quantity is in harmony with quality.

Chapter 3: Mastering Your Air Fryer

The Benefits of Air Frying Post-Surgery

In the dynamic world of culinary innovation, the air fryer stands out as a beacon of hope and possibility, especially for those navigating the new dietary realities post-gastric sleeve surgery. This remarkable appliance is more than a kitchen gadget; it's a partner in the journey towards a healthier, more vibrant life. Understanding the benefits of air frying post-surgery is crucial in harnessing its full potential to transform your eating habits.

1. Healthier Cooking Method

Post-gastric sleeve surgery, your dietary focus shifts towards healthier, nutrient-rich foods. The air fryer aligns perfectly with this goal. By using hot air to cook food, it minimizes the need for oil, drastically reducing the calorie and fat content of your meals. Traditional frying methods immerse food in oil, significantly increasing the fat and calorie content, which can be detrimental to your weight loss and health goals. The air fryer offers a way to enjoy the texture and flavor of fried foods without the health risks associated with deep frying.

2. Preserving Nutritional Value

Cooking methods can significantly impact the nutritional value of food. The air fryer excels in preserving vitamins and minerals that might be lost in other cooking methods like boiling or deep frying. By circulating hot air around the food, it cooks quickly and evenly, retaining the natural flavors and nutrients. This is particularly beneficial post-surgery when your body needs all the nutrients it can get for a speedy and effective recovery.

3. Versatility in Cooking

The versatility of the air fryer is a game-changer. It's not limited to frying; it can grill, roast, and even bake. This multifunctionality is invaluable when your diet needs variety but your energy and time for cooking might be limited. You can prepare a wide range of foods - from crispy vegetables and tender meats to baked goods and more - all with one appliance. This versatility helps keep your diet interesting and varied, which is essential for long-term adherence to a healthy eating plan.

4. Portion Control Made Easy

With its compact cooking space, the air fryer naturally lends itself to smaller portions, which is crucial in managing your new dietary requirements. The temptation to overeat is reduced when you cook in smaller batches. It allows for more controlled, mindful eating practices, which are essential after gastric sleeve surgery. The ability to cook single servings or small portions also means that you're always eating fresh, reducing the reliance on processed, pre-packaged foods.

5. Simplicity and Convenience

Post-surgery, your lifestyle might demand simplicity and convenience, especially in the kitchen. The air fryer is user-friendly, with straightforward settings and a hassle-free cleanup process, making it a practical choice for those who are new to cooking or those who find cooking a laborious task. Its quick cooking time also means you can prepare healthy meals even on your busiest days, supporting your dietary goals without adding stress.

6. Supporting Weight Management Goals

One of the primary goals post-gastric sleeve surgery is effective weight management. The air fryer supports this goal by providing a way to cook delicious, satisfying meals that are low in calories and fat. This method of cooking aligns with the dietary guidelines recommended for post-surgery patients, helping you maintain the progress you've made in your weight loss journey.

7. Emotional and Psychological Benefits

The benefits of the air fryer extend beyond the physical. There's an emotional and psychological component to cooking and eating. The ability to enjoy a variety of tasty, visually appealing foods that are also healthy can have a positive impact on your mood and overall well-being. It can reduce feelings of dietary restriction or deprivation, which are common post-surgery. The joy of cooking and eating plays a significant role in your recovery and adaptation to a new lifestyle.

Getting to Know Your Air Fryer

Embarking on a journey with your air fryer post-gastric sleeve surgery is an exploration into a new world of culinary possibilities. This versatile kitchen appliance, operating on the principles of rapid air technology, promises to be a cornerstone in your revamped, health-centric kitchen. Understanding its workings, capabilities, and maintenance is key to unlocking its full potential in your daily diet.

At its core, an air fryer circulates hot air around the food, creating a crispy layer reminiscent of traditional frying but without the hefty requirement of oil. This cooking method is not only healthier but also retains the taste and texture we often crave in fried foods. The essential components of an air fryer include the basket where you place the food, the tray that catches any drippings, and the main unit which houses the heating element and fan. Becoming familiar with these components is the first step in your air frying journey.

One of the most significant features of an air fryer is its ability to cook food at a precise temperature and for a set duration. This precision allows for consistent results, making it an invaluable tool for someone adapting to a new dietary lifestyle post-surgery. Most air fryers come equipped with adjustable temperature controls and timers, allowing for flexibility depending on the type of food being prepared. Learning how different foods react to varying temperatures and cooking times is an essential skill in mastering air fryer cooking.

A crucial step often overlooked in air frying is preheating. Much like a traditional oven, preheating your air fryer ensures that your food starts cooking immediately at the right temperature, crucial for achieving that perfect crispiness. Some models have a specific preheat setting, while others may

require running the air fryer empty for a few minutes at the cooking temperature.

Understanding spacing and the concept of batch cooking is another important aspect. Air frying requires sufficient space around each piece of food to facilitate proper air circulation, ensuring even cooking. This might mean cooking in smaller batches, but it guarantees that each piece is cooked to perfection. Regularly shaking the basket or flipping the food is also crucial in air frying. This practice helps to expose all sides of the food to the hot air, preventing uneven cooking.

Maintaining your air fryer is vital for both hygiene and the appliance's longevity. Regular cleaning prevents the buildup of food residues and odors. Most air fryers feature removable, non-stick baskets and trays that are dishwasher safe, simplifying the cleanup process.

Lastly, getting to know your air fryer is a journey of experimentation and adaptation. Each model has its unique characteristics, and starting with basic recipes before moving to more complex dishes is advisable. This allows you to understand how your specific model functions and how you can adapt traditional recipes to this new cooking method.

Tips and Tricks for Perfect Air Frying Every Time

As you embark on your post-gastric sleeve journey with your air fryer by your side, mastering its use can transform your daily cooking experiences. Here are some invaluable tips and tricks that will help you achieve perfect results with your air fryer, making each meal a delightful, healthy adventure.

1. Start with a Good Recipe: As you're getting familiar with your air fryer, begin with tried-and-tested recipes specifically designed for air frying. These recipes will guide you on the right temperatures and cooking times, taking much of the guesswork out of the equation.

2. Don't Overcrowd the Basket: Air fryers work by circulating hot air around the food. Overcrowding the basket hinders this process, leading to uneven cooking. Cook in batches if necessary, ensuring there's enough space for the air to circulate freely around each piece of food.

3. Shake or Turn Halfway Through: For evenly cooked food, shake the basket halfway through the cooking time or turn the food over. This simple step is crucial for foods like fries, vegetables, or smaller bites that need even exposure to the hot air.

4. Use Just a Touch of Oil: Although one of the air fryer's benefits is reducing the need for oil, a light spritz of cooking spray or a brush of oil can enhance the texture and flavor of certain foods. It helps achieve that golden, crispy exterior that makes air-fried foods so appealing.

5. Preheat for Best Results: Just like a conventional oven, preheating your air fryer can lead to better cooking results. A preheated air fryer ensures the food starts cooking immediately, crucial for getting that crispy texture.

6. Pat Foods Dry: Before cooking, especially items like chicken or potatoes, pat them dry. Removing excess moisture helps in achieving a crispier result, as the hot air can focus on browning and crisping rather than steaming.

7. Check Food Early and Often: Each air fryer model is different, and cooking times can vary. Start checking your food a few minutes before the recipe's suggested cooking time ends, especially if it's your first time preparing that dish in the air fryer.

8. Invest in Accessories: Accessories like parchment liners or grill pans designed for air fryers can enhance your cooking experience. They can help with easier clean-up and allow for more versatility in the types of dishes you can prepare.

9. Keep It Clean: Regular cleaning is not just about maintenance; it also affects cooking performance. Built-up grease and food particles can alter how food cooks and tastes. Clean your air fryer after each use to keep it functioning optimally.

10. Be Creative and Experiment: Once you're comfortable with the basics, start experimenting. Try different foods and recipes. The air fryer's versatility extends from appetizers to desserts, so don't hesitate to explore its full potential.

11. Stay Safe: Always use oven mitts when handling the hot basket, and be cautious of steam when opening the air fryer after cooking. Ensure your air fryer is placed on a heat-resistant, stable surface and not near any flammable objects.

Embracing these tips and tricks will elevate your air frying experience, making every meal an opportunity to enjoy healthy, delicious, and perfectly cooked food.

Chapter 4: Recipes

Phase 1: Liquid Diet Recipes - Nourishing Broths

Golden Turmeric Bone Broth

- P.T.: 3 hours
- Ingr.: 2 lbs beef bones, 1 onion (chopped), 2 carrots (chopped), 1 tbsp turmeric, 2 cloves garlic (minced), 6 cups water.
- Process: Roast bones in air fryer at 400°F for 20 mins. Simmer with all ingredients in a pot for 3 hours. Strain.
- Shopping list: Beef bones, onion, carrots, turmeric, garlic.
- N.I.: Calories: 40, Protein: 6g, Fat: 2g, Carbs: 3g.

Healing Ginger Chicken Broth

- P.T.: 3 hours
- Ingr.: 1 lb chicken bones, 1-inch ginger (sliced), 1 onion (quartered), 6 cups water, 1 stalk celery (chopped).
- Process: Air fry chicken bones and ginger at 375°F for 15 mins. Simmer in pot with other ingredients for 3 hours. Strain.
- Shopping list: Chicken bones, ginger, onion, celery.

- N.I.: Calories: 35, Protein: 5g, Fat: 1g,
- Carbs: 2g.

Soothing Lemongrass Beef Broth

- P.T.: 3 hours
- Ingr.: 2 lbs beef bones, 2 stalks lemongrass (crushed), 1 onion (chopped), 6 cups water, 1 bay leaf.
- Process: Air fry beef bones and lemongrass at 400°F for 20 mins. Simmer with remaining ingredients for 3 hours. Strain.
- Shopping list: Beef bones, lemongrass, onion, bay leaf.

- N.I.: Calories: 45, Protein: 7g, Fat: 2g, Carbs: 3g.

Mint and Lamb Healing Broth

- P.T.: 3 hours
- Ingr.: 1.5 lbs lamb bones, 6 cups water, 1 onion (quartered), 1/2 cup fresh mint, 1 carrot (chopped).

- Process: Air fry lamb bones at 375°F for 20 mins. Simmer with all ingredients for 3 hours. Strain.
- Shopping list: Lamb bones, mint, onion, carrot.

- N.I.: Calories: 50, Carbs: 4g.
  Protein: 8g, Fat: 3g,

Citrus-Infused Fish Broth

- P.T.: 2 hours
- Ingr.: 2 lbs fish bones, 6 cups water, 1 lemon (sliced), 1 onion (chopped), 1 tsp peppercorns.
- Process: Air fry fish bones at 350°F for 15 mins. Simmer with other ingredients for 2 hours. Strain.
- Shopping list: Fish bones, lemon, onion, peppercorns.
- N.I.: Calories: 30, Protein: 6g, Fat: 1g, Carbs: 2g.

Spicy Tomato and Bone Broth

- P.T.: 3 hours
- Ingr.: 2 lbs mixed bones, 6 cups water, 1 cup tomato puree, 1 tsp chili flakes, 1 onion (chopped).
- Process: Air fry bones at 400°F for 20 mins. Simmer with all ingredients for 3 hours. Strain.
- Shopping list: Mixed bones, tomato puree, chili flakes, onion.
- N.I.: Calories: 50, Protein: 8g, Fat: 2g, Carbs: 4g.

Herbal Turkey Broth

- P.T.: 3 hours
- Ingr.: 2 lbs turkey bones, 6 cups water, 1 cup fresh parsley, 1 onion (chopped), 2 carrots (chopped).
- Process: Air fry turkey bones at 375°F for 20 mins. Simmer with other ingredients for 3 hours. Strain.
- Shopping list: Turkey bones, parsley, onion, carrots.
- N.I.: Calories: 40, Protein: 6g, Fat: 2g, Carbs: 3g.

Asian-Style Pork Broth

- P.T.: 3 hours
- Ingr.: 2 lbs pork bones, 6 cups water, 2 star anise, 1 inch ginger (sliced), 1 onion (chopped).
- Process: Air fry pork bones and ginger at 375°F for 20 mins. Simmer with star anise and onion for 3 hours. Strain.
- Shopping list: Pork bones, star anise, ginger, onion.
- N.I.: Calories: 45, Protein: 7g, Fat: 3g, Carbs: 4g.

Rosemary and Veal Bone Broth

- P.T.: 3 hours
- Ingr.: 2 lbs veal bones, 6 cups water, 1 sprig rosemary, 1 onion (chopped), 2 cloves garlic (minced).
- Process: Air fry veal bones at 375°F for 20 mins. Simmer with other ingredients for 3 hours. Strain.

- Shopping list: Veal bones, rosemary, onion, garlic.
- N.I.: Calories: 50, Protein: 8g, Fat: 3g, Carbs: 3g.

Zingy Pepper and Chicken Broth

- P.T.: 3 hours
- Ingr.: 2 lbs chicken bones, 6 cups water, 1 red bell pepper (chopped), 1 onion (chopped), 1 tsp black pepper.
- Process: Air fry chicken bones at 375°F for 20 mins. Simmer with all ingredients for 3 hours. Strain.

- Shopping list: Chicken bones, red bell pepper, onion, black pepper.
- N.I.: Calories: 35, Protein: 6g, Fat: 1g, Carbs: 4g.

Cilantro Lime Seafood Broth

- P.T.: 2 hours
- Ingr.: 2 lbs seafood shells, 6 cups water, 1 cup fresh cilantro, juice of 1 lime, 1 onion (chopped).
- Process: Air fry seafood shells at 350°F for 15 mins. Simmer with other ingredients for 2 hours. Strain.
- Shopping list: Seafood shells, cilantro, lime, onion.
- N.I.: Calories: 30, Protein: 5g, Fat: 1g, Carbs: 3g.

Earthy Mushroom and Garlic Broth

- P.T.: 3 hours
- Ingr.: 1 lb mixed mushrooms, 6 cups water, 4 cloves garlic (minced), 1 onion (chopped), 1 tsp thyme.
- Process: Air fry mushrooms and garlic at 375°F for 15 mins. Simmer with thyme and onion for 3 hours. Strain.
- Shopping list: Mixed mushrooms, garlic, onion, thyme.
- N.I.: Calories: 40, Protein: 4g, Fat: 1g, Carbs: 8g.

Soothing Carrot and Ginger Broth

- P.T.: 3 hours
- Ingr.: 1 lb chicken bones, 6 cups water, 2 carrots (chopped), 1-inch ginger (sliced), 1 onion (chopped).
- Process: Air fry chicken bones and ginger at 375°F for 20 mins. Simmer with carrots and onion for 3 hours. Strain.
- Shopping list: Chicken bones, carrots, ginger, onion.
- N.I.: Calories: 35, Protein: 5g, Fat: 1g, Carbs: 5g.

Invigorating Peppermint and Lamb Broth

- P.T.: 3 hours
- Ingr.: 2 lbs lamb bones, 6 cups water, ½ cup fresh peppermint leaves, 1 onion (chopped), 2 cloves garlic (minced).
- Process: Air fry lamb bones at 375°F for 20 mins. Simmer with peppermint, garlic, and onion for 3 hours. Strain.
- Shopping list: Lamb bones, peppermint leaves, onion, garlic.
- N.I.: Calories: 50, Protein: 8g, Fat: 3g, Carbs: 4g.

Ginger Infused Chicken Broth

- P.T.: 3 hrs
- Ingr.: 2 lbs chicken bones, 1-inch ginger, 1 onion, 6 cups water, salt.
- Process: Simmer chicken bones, ginger, onion, and salt in water for 3 hrs. Strain.

- Shopping list: Chicken bones, ginger, onion.
- N.I.: Calories: 50, Protein: 8g, Fat: 2g, Carbs: 3g.

Nutritious Smoothies and Juices

Antioxidant Berry Blast Smoothie

- P.T.: 5 mins
- Ingr.: 1 cup mixed berries (frozen), 1 banana, 1 cup spinach, 1 cup almond milk.
- Process: Blend all ingredients until smooth.

- Shopping list: Mixed berries, banana, spinach, almond milk.
- N.I.: Calories: 180, Protein: 4g, Fat: 3g, Carbs: 35g.

Green Detox Juice

- P.T.: 10 mins
- Ingr.: 2 cups kale, 1 green apple, 1 cucumber, 1 lemon (juiced), 1-inch ginger.
- Process: Juice all ingredients.

- Shopping list: Kale, green apple, cucumber, lemon, ginger.
- N.I.: Calories: 120, Protein: 3g, Fat: 1g, Carbs: 28g.

Tropical Mango Smoothie

- P.T.: 5 mins
- Ingr.: 1 cup mango (frozen), 1 banana, 1 cup coconut water, 1 tbsp flaxseed.
- Process: Blend all ingredients until smooth.

- Shopping list: Mango, banana, coconut water, flaxseed.
- N.I.: Calories: 200, Protein: 3g, Fat: 2g, Carbs: 45g.

Soothing Almond Milk and Vanilla Shake

- P.T.: 5 mins
- Ingr.: 1 cup almond milk, 1 tsp vanilla extract, 1 tbsp almond butter, 1 tsp honey.
- Process: Blend all ingredients until smooth.
- Shopping list: Almond milk, vanilla extract, almond butter, honey.
- N.I.: Calories: 150, Protein: 3g, Fat: 9g, Carbs: 15g.

Red Beet and Berry Juice

- P.T.: 10 mins
- Ingr.: 1 beet (peeled), 1 cup strawberries, 1 carrot, 1 orange (juiced).
- Process: Juice all ingredients.
- Shopping list: Beet, strawberries, carrot, orange.
- N.I.: Calories: 140, Protein: 2g, Fat: 1g, Carbs: 32g.

Carrot and Ginger Zinger Juice

- P.T.: 10 mins
- Ingr.: 4 carrots, 1-inch ginger, 1 lemon (juiced), 1 apple.
- Process: Juice all ingredients.
- Shopping list: Carrots, ginger, lemon, apple.
- N.I.: Calories: 120, Protein: 2g, Fat: 1g, Carbs: 28g.

Creamy Avocado and Spinach Smoothie

- P.T.: 5 mins
- Ingr.: ½ avocado, 1 cup spinach, 1 cup Greek yogurt, 1 tsp honey.
- Process: Blend all ingredients until smooth.
- Shopping list: Avocado, spinach, Greek yogurt, honey.
- N.I.: Calories: 220, Protein: 12g, Fat: 12g, Carbs: 20g.

Blueberry Oatmeal Breakfast Smoothie

- P.T.: 5 mins
- Ingr.: 1 cup blueberries (frozen), ½ cup rolled oats, 1 cup almond milk, 1 tbsp almond butter.
- Process: Blend all ingredients until smooth.
- Shopping list: Blueberries, rolled oats, almond milk, almond butter.
- N.I.: Calories: 250, Protein: 6g, Fat: 9g, Carbs: 38g.

Refreshing Cucumber and Lime Juice

- P.T.: 10 mins
- Ingr.: 2 cucumbers, 2 limes (juiced), 1 cup water, mint leaves.
- Process: Juice cucumbers and limes, mix with water, garnish with mint.
- Shopping list: Cucumbers, limes, mint.
- N.I.: Calories: 50, Protein: 2g, Fat: 0g, Carbs: 12g.

Pineapple and Ginger Immune Booster

- P.T.: 10 mins
- Ingr.: 1 cup pineapple, 1-inch ginger, 1 orange (juiced), 1 carrot.
- Process: Juice all ingredients.

- Shopping list: Pineapple, ginger, orange, carrot.
- N.I.: Calories: 130, Protein: 2g, Fat: 1g, Carbs: 30g.

Protein-Packed Chocolate Almond Shake

- P.T.: 5 mins
- Ingr.: 1 cup almond milk, 1 scoop chocolate protein powder, 1 tbsp almond butter, ice cubes.
- Process: Blend all ingredients until smooth.

- Shopping list: Almond milk, chocolate protein powder, almond butter.
- N.I.: Calories: 250, Protein: 20g, Fat: 12g, Carbs: 15g.

Vibrant Veggie Green Juice

- P.T.: 10 mins
- Ingr.: 2 cups spinach, 1 green apple, 1 cucumber, 1 celery stalk, 1 lemon (juiced).
- Process: Juice all ingredients.

- Shopping list: Spinach, green apple, cucumber, celery, lemon.
- N.I.: Calories: 100, Protein: 3g, Fat: 1g, Carbs: 22g.

Golden Milk Turmeric Smoothie

- P.T.: 5 mins
- Ingr.: 1 cup almond milk, 1 tsp turmeric, 1 banana, 1 tsp honey, pinch of black pepper.
- Process: Blend all ingredients until smooth.
- Shopping list: Almond milk, turmeric, banana, honey, black pepper.
- N.I.: Calories: 150, Protein: 2g, Fat: 3g, Carbs: 30g.

Spiced Apple Cinnamon Juice

- P.T.: 10 mins
- Ingr.: 2 apples, 1 cinnamon stick, 1 cup water, 1 tsp honey.
- Process: Juice apples, simmer with cinnamon stick and water, add honey.
- Shopping list: Apples, cinnamon stick, honey.
- N.I.: Calories: 110, Protein: 0g, Fat: 0g, Carbs: 28g.

Strawberry Kiwi Hydration Smoothie

- P.T.: 5 mins
- Ingr.: 1 cup strawberries, 2 kiwis (peeled), 1 cup coconut water, 1 tbsp chia seeds.
- Process: Blend all ingredients until smooth.
- Shopping list: Strawberries, kiwis, coconut water, chia seeds.
- N.I.: Calories: 180, Protein: 4g, Fat: 4g, Carbs: 35g.

Phase 2: Pureed and Soft Foods - Pureed Vegetables

Roasted Carrot and Ginger Puree

- P.T.: 40 mins
- Ingr.: 4 large carrots (chopped), 1-inch ginger (grated), 2 tbsp olive oil, salt.
- Process: Roast carrots and ginger with olive oil in the air fryer at 360°F for 20-25 minutes until tender.

Blend until smooth.
- Shopping list: Carrots, ginger, olive oil.
- N.I.: Calories: 90, Protein: 1g, Fat: 7g, Carbs: 8g.

Creamy Broccoli and Avocado Blend

- P.T.: 25 mins
- Ingr.: 2 cups broccoli florets, ½ ripe avocado, 1 tbsp Greek yogurt, salt, pepper.
- Process: Air fry broccoli florets with a bit of oil at 360°F for 8-10 minutes.

Blend with avocado and Greek yogurt.
- Shopping list: Broccoli, avocado, Greek yogurt.
- N.I.: Calories: 100, Protein: 4g, Fat: 6g, Carbs: 9g.

Pumpkin and White Bean Mousse

- P.T.: 30 mins
- Ingr.: 1 cup pumpkin puree, ½ cup canned white beans, 1 tsp cinnamon, 1 tbsp maple syrup.
- Process: Blend pumpkin, beans, cinnamon, and maple syrup until creamy.
- Shopping list: Pumpkin puree, white beans, cinnamon, maple syrup.
- N.I.: Calories: 120, Protein: 3g, Fat: 0.5g, Carbs: 25g.

Smooth Zucchini and Basil Blend

- P.T.: 20 mins
- Ingr.: 3 zucchinis (chopped), ¼ cup fresh basil, 1 tbsp olive oil, salt, pepper.
- Process: Air fry chopped zucchini with olive oil at 360°F for 10-15 minutes. Blend with basil, olive oil, salt, and pepper.
- Shopping list: Zucchinis, basil, olive oil.
- N.I.: Calories: 60, Protein: 2g, Fat: 5g, Carbs: 4g.

Velvety Beet and Yogurt Puree

- P.T.: 45 mins
- Ingr.: 2 medium beets (cubed), ½ cup Greek yogurt, 1 tsp honey, salt.
- Process: Wrap beets in foil and air fry at 360°F for 30-35 minutes. Once cooled, blend with Greek yogurt, honey, and salt.
- Shopping list: Beets, Greek yogurt, honey.
- N.I.: Calories: 100, Protein: 5g, Fat: 1g, Carbs: 18g.

Cauliflower and Chive Cream

- P.T.: 25 mins
- Ingr.: 1 head cauliflower (chopped), 2 tbsp chives (chopped), 1 tbsp cream cheese, salt, pepper.
- Process: Air fry chopped cauliflower with a bit of oil at 360°F for 15-20 minutes. Blend with chives and cream cheese.
- Shopping list: Cauliflower, chives, cream cheese.
- N.I.: Calories: 70, Protein: 3g, Fat: 3g, Carbs: 9g.

Sweet Potato and Cinnamon Mash

- P.T.: 35 mins
- Ingr.: 2 sweet potatoes (peeled, cubed), 1 tsp cinnamon, 1 tbsp almond milk, salt.
- Process: Air fry cubed sweet potatoes at 360°F for 20-25 minutes.

Mash with cinnamon and almond milk.

- Shopping list: Sweet potatoes, cinnamon, almond milk.
- N.I.: Calories: 110, Protein: 2g, Fat: 1g, Carbs: 24g.

Savory Lentil and Carrot Cream

- P.T.: 40 mins
- Ingr.: 1 cup red lentils, 2 carrots (chopped), 1 tsp cumin, salt, pepper.
- Process: Air fry chopped carrots at 360°F for 15-20 minutes.

Cook lentils separately and blend with roasted carrots, cumin, salt, and pepper.

- Shopping list: Red lentils, carrots, cumin.
- N.I.: Calories: 120, Protein: 7g, Fat: 0.5g, Carbs: 20g.

Pea and Mint Puree

- P.T.: 15 mins
- Ingr.: 1 cup frozen peas, 2 tbsp fresh mint, 1 tbsp olive oil, salt.
- Process: Air fry frozen peas for about 5-7 minutes.

Blend with mint, olive oil, and salt.

- Shopping list: Frozen peas, mint, olive oil.
- N.I.: Calories: 100, Protein: 5g, Fat: 4g, Carbs: 12g.

Roasted Red Pepper and Walnut Spread

- P.T.: 30 mins
- Ingr.: 2 red bell peppers, ½ cup walnuts, 1 garlic clove, 1 tbsp olive oil, salt, pepper.
- Process: Air fry red bell peppers at 360°F for 15-20 minutes. Blend with walnuts, garlic, olive oil, salt, and pepper.
- Shopping list: Red bell peppers, walnuts, garlic, olive oil.
- N.I.: Calories: 150, Protein: 4g, Fat: 12g, Carbs: 9g.

Soft and Creamy Breakfast Options

Apple Cinnamon Oatmeal Puree

- P.T.: 15 mins
- Ingr.: ½ cup rolled oats, 1 apple (peeled and pureed), 1 cup almond milk, ½ tsp cinnamon, 1 tsp honey.
- Process: Air fry chopped apple with a sprinkle of cinnamon at 360°F for 10-12 minutes. Cook oats in almond milk and blend with roasted apple.
- Shopping list: Rolled oats, apple, almond milk, cinnamon, honey.
- N.I.: Calories: 180, Protein: 5g, Fat: 3g, Carbs: 35g.

Berry Yogurt Bliss

- P.T.: 10 mins
- Ingr.: 1 cup Greek yogurt, ½ cup mixed berries (pureed), 1 tbsp honey, 1 tsp chia seeds.
- Process: Mix yogurt with berry puree, honey, and chia seeds.
- Shopping list: Greek yogurt, mixed berries, honey, chia seeds.
- N.I.: Calories: 200, Protein: 15g, Fat: 3g, Carbs: 30g.

Creamy Avocado and Banana Smoothie

- P.T.: 5 mins
- Ingr.: 1 ripe avocado, 1 banana, 1 cup almond milk, 1 tbsp honey.
- Process: Blend avocado, banana, almond milk, and honey until smooth.
- Shopping list: Avocado, banana, almond milk, honey.
- N.I.: Calories: 250, Protein: 5g, Fat: 15g, Carbs: 28g.

Peaches and Cream Oatmeal

- P.T.: 20 mins
- Ingr.: ½ cup rolled oats, 1 cup almond milk, 1 peach (pureed), 1 tsp vanilla extract, 1 tsp honey.
- Process: Air fry chopped peach with a bit of honey at 360°F for 10-12 minutes. Cook oats with almond milk, then blend with roasted peach.
- Shopping list: Rolled oats, almond milk, peach, vanilla extract, honey.
- N.I.: Calories: 190, Protein: 6g, Fat: 3g, Carbs: 35g.

Silken Tofu and Berry Pudding

- P.T.: 10 mins
- Ingr.: 1 cup silken tofu, ½ cup mixed berries, 1 tbsp maple syrup, 1 tsp lemon juice.
- Process: Blend tofu, berries, maple syrup, and lemon juice until smooth.
- Shopping list: Silken tofu, mixed berries, maple syrup, lemon.
- N.I.: Calories: 150, Protein: 8g, Fat: 5g, Carbs: 20g.

Mango Coconut Rice Pudding

- P.T.: 25 mins
- Ingr.: ½ cup cooked rice, 1 cup coconut milk, 1 mango (pureed), 1 tsp honey, ½ tsp cinnamon.
- Process: Air fry cubed mango at 360°F for 8-10 minutes. Mix with cooked rice, coconut milk, honey, and cinnamon.
- Shopping list: Rice, coconut milk, mango, honey, cinnamon.
- N.I.: Calories: 200, Protein: 3g, Fat: 7g, Carbs: 35g.

Pumpkin Spice Smoothie

- P.T.: 10 mins
- Ingr.: ½ cup pumpkin puree, 1 cup almond milk, 1 banana, 1 tsp pumpkin spice, 1 tbsp maple syrup.
- Process: Blend pumpkin puree, almond milk, banana, pumpkin spice, and maple syrup.
- Shopping list: Pumpkin puree, almond milk, banana, pumpkin spice, maple syrup.
- N.I.: Calories: 210, Protein: 4g, Fat: 3g, Carbs: 45g.

Almond Butter and Jelly Oatmeal

- P.T.: 15 mins
- Ingr.: ½ cup rolled oats, 1 cup almond milk, 2 tbsp almond butter, 2 tbsp strawberry puree, 1 tsp honey.
- Process: Air fry strawberry puree at 360°F for 5-7 minutes to intensify flavor. Cook oats with almond milk and blend with almond butter and roasted strawberry puree.
- Shopping list: Rolled oats, almond milk, almond butter, strawberries, honey.
- N.I.: Calories: 250, Protein: 8g, Fat: 12g, Carbs: 30g.

Cinnamon Apple Quinoa Porridge

- P.T.: 20 mins
- Ingr.: ½ cup quinoa, 1 cup almond milk, 1 apple (peeled and pureed), ½ tsp cinnamon, 1 tsp honey.
- Process: Air fry chopped apple with cinnamon at 360°F for 10-12 minutes.

Cook quinoa in almond milk and blend with roasted apple.

- Shopping list: Quinoa, almond milk, apple, cinnamon, honey.
- N.I.: Calories: 200, Protein: 6g, Fat: 3g, Carbs: 38g.

Sweet Potato and Maple Mash

- P.T.: 30 mins
- Ingr.: 1 large sweet potato (cooked and mashed), 2 tbsp almond milk, 1 tbsp maple syrup, ½ tsp cinnamon.
- Process: Air fry whole sweet potato at 360°F for 30-35 minutes.

Mash with almond milk, maple syrup, and cinnamon.

- Shopping list: Sweet potato, almond milk, maple syrup, cinnamon.
- N.I.: Calories: 150, Protein: 2g, Fat: 1g, Carbs: 35g.

Gentle Snacks and Appetizers

Carrot and Coriander Soup

- P.T.: 30 mins
- Ingr.: 4 carrots (peeled, chopped), 1 onion (chopped), 2 cups vegetable broth, 1 tsp ground coriander, salt, pepper.
- Process: Air fry chopped carrots and onion with a bit of oil at 360°F for 15 minutes. Simmer in vegetable broth with coriander, then blend.
- Shopping list: Carrots, onion, vegetable broth, ground coriander.
- N.I.: Calories: 70, Protein: 2g, Fat: 0.5g, Carbs: 16g.

Creamy Avocado Dip

- P.T.: 10 mins
- Ingr.: 1 ripe avocado, 1 tbsp Greek yogurt, 1 tsp lemon juice, salt, pepper.
- Process: Mash avocado, mix with yogurt, lemon juice, salt, and pepper.
- Shopping list: Avocado, Greek yogurt, lemon.
- N.I.: Calories: 120, Protein: 3g, Fat: 10g, Carbs: 8g.

Mashed Pea and Mint Spread

- P.T.: 20 mins
- Ingr.: 1 cup frozen peas, 2 tbsp fresh mint (chopped), 1 tbsp olive oil, salt, pepper.
- Process: Air fry frozen peas for 5-7 minutes. Blend with mint, olive oil, salt, and pepper.
- Shopping list: Frozen peas, fresh mint, olive oil.
- N.I.: Calories: 100, Protein: 4g, Fat: 5g, Carbs: 10g.

Roasted Red Pepper Hummus

- P.T.: 15 mins
- Ingr.: 1 cup canned chickpeas (drained), 1 roasted red pepper, 1 garlic clove, 1 tbsp tahini, lemon juice, salt.
- Process: Air fry red pepper at 360°F for 15-20 minutes, then blend with chickpeas, garlic, tahini, and lemon juice.
- Shopping list: Chickpeas, red pepper, garlic, tahini.
- N.I.: Calories: 90, Protein: 4g, Fat: 3g, Carbs: 13g.

Baked Apple and Cinnamon Puree

- P.T.: 25 mins
- Ingr.: 2 apples (peeled, cored), ½ tsp cinnamon, 1 tsp honey, ¼ cup water.
- Process:
- Air fry apple slices with cinnamon and honey at 350°F for 10-15 minutes, then blend.
- Shopping list: Apples, cinnamon, honey.
- N.I.: Calories: 100, Protein: 0g, Fat: 0g, Carbs: 26g.

Sweet Potato and Ginger Soup

- P.T.: 35 mins
- Ingr.: 2 sweet potatoes (peeled, cubed), 1-inch ginger (minced), 2 cups vegetable broth, salt, pepper.
- Process: Air fry cubed sweet potatoes and minced ginger at 360°F for 20-25 minutes. Simmer in broth, then blend.
- Shopping list: Sweet potatoes, ginger, vegetable broth.
- N.I.: Calories: 120, Protein: 2g, Fat: 0.5g, Carbs: 28g.

Pumpkin and Nutmeg Mousse

- P.T.: 20 mins
- Ingr.: 1 cup pumpkin puree, ¼ cup Greek yogurt, 1 tsp nutmeg, 1 tbsp maple syrup.
- Process: Blend pumpkin puree, yogurt, nutmeg, and maple syrup until creamy.
- Shopping list: Pumpkin puree, Greek yogurt, nutmeg, maple syrup.
- N.I.: Calories: 100, Protein: 3g, Fat: 1g, Carbs: 20g.

Creamy Beet and Feta Dip

- P.T.: 40 mins
- Ingr.: 2 beets (cooked, peeled), ¼ cup feta cheese, 1 tbsp olive oil, lemon juice, salt.
- Process: Air fry whole beets wrapped in foil at 360°F for 30-35 minutes. Blend with feta, olive oil, lemon juice, and salt.
- Shopping list: Beets, feta cheese, olive oil, lemon.
- N.I.: Calories: 110, Protein: 3g, Fat: 7g, Carbs: 10g.

Zucchini and Basil Velouté

- P.T.: 25 mins
- Ingr.: 2 zucchinis (chopped), 1 cup vegetable broth, ¼ cup fresh basil, 1 tbsp cream, salt, pepper.
- Process: Air fry chopped zucchini at 360°F for 10-15 minutes. Simmer in broth with basil, add cream, then blend.
- Shopping list: Zucchinis, vegetable broth, basil, cream.
- N.I.: Calories: 60, Protein: 2g, Fat: 4g, Carbs: 6g.

Cauliflower and Parmesan Cream

- P.T.: 30 mins
- Ingr.: 1 head cauliflower (chopped), ¼ cup grated Parmesan, 1 tbsp cream, salt, pepper.
- Process: Air fry chopped cauliflower at 360°F for 15-20 minutes. Blend with Parmesan, cream, salt, and pepper.
- Shopping list: Cauliflower, Parmesan cheese, cream.
- N.I.: Calories: 100, Protein: 5g, Fat: 6g, Carbs: 8g.

Phase 3: Transition to Solid Foods - Poultry and Meat

Herb-Infused Chicken Breast

- P.T.: 25 mins
- Ingr.: 2 chicken breasts, 1 tsp thyme, 1 tsp rosemary, salt, pepper, olive oil spray.
- Process: Season chicken with herbs, salt, pepper. Spray with oil. Air fry at 360°F for 20 mins.
- Shopping list: Chicken breasts, thyme, rosemary, olive oil spray.
- N.I.: Calories: 165, Protein: 31g, Fat: 3g, Carbs: 0g.

Lemon Garlic Turkey Tenderloin

- P.T.: 30 mins
- Ingr.: 1 turkey tenderloin, 1 tbsp lemon juice, 1 garlic clove (minced), salt, pepper, olive oil spray.
- Process: Marinate turkey in lemon, garlic, salt, pepper. Spray with oil. Air fry at 360°F for 25 mins.
- Shopping list: Turkey tenderloin, lemon, garlic, olive oil spray.
- N.I.: Calories: 120, Protein: 26g, Fat: 1g, Carbs: 2g.

Spiced Ground Chicken Patties

- P.T.: 20 mins
- Ingr.: 1 lb ground chicken, 1 tsp paprika, ½ tsp cumin, salt, pepper, olive oil spray.
- Process: Mix chicken with spices. Form patties. Spray with oil. Air fry at 360°F for 15 mins.

- Shopping list: Ground chicken, paprika, cumin, olive oil spray.
- N.I.: Calories: 160, Protein: 22g, Fat: 8g, Carbs: 1g.

Rosemary and Thyme Turkey Meatballs

- P.T.: 25 mins
- Ingr.: 1 lb ground turkey, 1 tsp rosemary, 1 tsp thyme, salt, pepper, 1 egg.
- Process: Combine ingredients. Form meatballs. Air fry at 360°F for 20 mins.

- Shopping list: Ground turkey, rosemary, thyme, egg.
- N.I.: Calories: 140, Protein: 20g, Fat: 6g, Carbs: 2g.

Tender BBQ Chicken Thighs

- P.T.: 30 mins
- Ingr.: 4 chicken thighs, 2 tbsp BBQ sauce (low sugar), salt, pepper, olive oil spray.
- Process: Season thighs, brush with BBQ sauce. Spray with oil. Air fry at 360°F for 25 mins.
- Shopping list: Chicken thighs, BBQ sauce, olive oil spray.
- N.I.: Calories: 210, Protein: 18g, Fat: 14g, Carbs: 5g.

Garlic Herb Roasted Turkey Breast

- P.T.: 35 mins
- Ingr.: 1 turkey breast, 1 tsp garlic powder, 1 tsp mixed herbs, salt, pepper, olive oil spray.
- Process: Season turkey. Spray with oil. Air fry at 340°F for 30 mins.
- Shopping list: Turkey breast, garlic powder, mixed herbs, olive oil spray.
- N.I.: Calories: 125, Protein: 26g, Fat: 2g, Carbs: 1g.

Balsamic Glazed Chicken Drumsticks

- P.T.: 40 mins
- Ingr.: 6 chicken drumsticks, 2 tbsp balsamic vinegar, 1 tbsp honey, salt, pepper, olive oil spray.
- Process: Marinate drumsticks in vinegar, honey, salt, pepper. Spray with oil. Air fry at 360°F for 35 mins.
- Shopping list: Chicken drumsticks, balsamic vinegar, honey, olive oil spray.
- N.I.: Calories: 200, Protein: 24g, Fat: 10g, Carbs: 7g.

Simple Lemon Pepper Chicken Wings

- P.T.: 30 mins
- Ingr.: 1 lb chicken wings, 1 tbsp lemon pepper seasoning, olive oil spray.
- Process: Season wings with lemon pepper. Spray with oil. Air fry at 400°F for 25 mins.
- Shopping list: Chicken wings, lemon pepper seasoning, olive oil spray.
- N.I.: Calories: 190, Protein: 15g, Fat: 14g, Carbs: 1g.

Soy Glazed Turkey Meatloaf

- P.T.: 45 mins
- Ingr.: 1 lb ground turkey, 1 egg, ¼ cup breadcrumbs (gluten-free), 2 tbsp soy sauce, 1 tsp garlic powder, salt, pepper.
- Process: Mix ingredients. Form loaf. Air fry at 360°F for 40 mins. Glaze with extra soy sauce.
- Shopping list: Ground turkey, egg, breadcrumbs, soy sauce, garlic powder.
- N.I.: Calories: 180, Protein: 25g, Fat: 8g, Carbs: 5g.

Honey Mustard Chicken Tenders

- P.T.: 25 mins
- Ingr.: 1 lb chicken tenders, 2 tbsp honey mustard sauce, salt, pepper, olive oil spray.
- Process: Season tenders with salt, pepper. Coat with sauce. Spray with oil. Air fry at 360°F for 20 mins.
- Shopping list: Chicken tenders, honey mustard sauce, olive oil spray.
- N.I.: Calories: 165, Protein: 25g, Fat: 4g, Carbs: 7g.

Fish & Seafood

Lemon Herb Air-Fried Salmon

- P.T.: 20 mins
- Ingr.: 2 salmon fillets, 1 tbsp lemon juice, 1 tsp dried dill, salt, pepper, olive oil spray.
- Process: Season salmon with lemon juice, dill, salt, pepper. Spray with oil. Air fry at 360°F for 12 mins.
- Shopping list: Salmon fillets, lemon juice, dried dill, olive oil spray.
- N.I.: Calories: 200, Protein: 23g, Fat: 12g, Carbs: 1g.

Garlic Butter Air-Fried Shrimp

- P.T.: 15 mins
- Ingr.: 1 lb shrimp (peeled, deveined), 2 tbsp butter (melted), 1 garlic clove (minced), parsley, salt, pepper.
- Process: Toss shrimp in butter, garlic, parsley, salt, pepper. Air fry at 370°F for 10 mins.
- Shopping list: Shrimp, butter, garlic, parsley.
- N.I.: Calories: 150, Protein: 24g, Fat: 6g, Carbs: 1g.

Crispy Air-Fried Tilapia

- P.T.: 20 mins
- Ingr.: 2 tilapia fillets, 1 egg (beaten), ½ cup breadcrumbs, 1 tsp paprika, salt, pepper, olive oil spray.
- Process: Dip fillets in egg, coat in breadcrumbs mixed with paprika, salt, pepper. Spray with oil. Air fry at 380°F for 15 mins.
- Shopping list: Tilapia fillets, egg, breadcrumbs, paprika, olive oil spray.
- N.I.: Calories: 210, Protein: 28g, Fat: 7g, Carbs: 9g.

Spiced Cod Air-Fryer Delight

- P.T.: 22 mins
- Ingr.: 2 cod fillets, 1 tsp chili powder, ½ tsp cumin, salt, pepper, olive oil spray.
- Process: Season cod with chili powder, cumin, salt, pepper. Spray with oil. Air fry at 360°F for 12 mins.
- Shopping list: Cod fillets, chili powder, cumin, olive oil spray.
- N.I.: Calories: 120, Protein: 20g, Fat: 3g, Carbs: 1g.

Herbed Shrimp and Asparagus

- P.T.: 18 mins
- Ingr.: 1 lb shrimp, 1 bunch asparagus (trimmed), 1 tsp Italian seasoning, lemon zest, salt, pepper, olive oil spray.
- Process: Toss shrimp, asparagus with seasoning, zest, salt, pepper. Spray with oil. Air fry at 370°F for 15 mins.
- Shopping list: Shrimp, asparagus, Italian seasoning, lemon, olive oil spray.
- N.I.: Calories: 160, Protein: 25g, Fat: 4g, Carbs: 5g.

Air-Fried Flounder with Lemon Pepper

- P.T.: 20 mins
- Ingr.: 2 flounder fillets, 1 tbsp lemon pepper seasoning, salt, olive oil spray.
- Process: Season fillets with lemon pepper, salt. Spray with oil. Air fry at 360°F for 10 mins.
- Shopping list: Flounder fillets, lemon pepper seasoning, olive oil spray.
- N.I.: Calories: 120, Protein: 20g, Fat: 3g, Carbs: 1g.

Simple Air-Fried Scallops

- P.T.: 12 mins
- Ingr.: 1 lb scallops, salt, pepper, 1 tbsp lemon juice, olive oil spray.
- Process: Season scallops with salt, pepper, lemon juice. Spray with oil. Air fry at 400°F for 10 mins.

- Shopping list: Scallops, lemon juice, olive oil spray.
- N.I.: Calories: 100, Protein: 20g, Fat: 1g, Carbs: 3g.

Lime Cilantro Air-Fried Haddock

- P.T.: 18 mins
- Ingr.: 2 haddock fillets, 1 tbsp lime juice, 1 tsp cilantro (chopped), salt, pepper, olive oil spray.
- Process: Season haddock with lime juice, cilantro, salt, pepper. Spray with oil. Air fry at 360°F for 15 mins.

- Shopping list: Haddock fillets, lime juice, cilantro, olive oil spray.
- N.I.: Calories: 120, Protein: 20g, Fat: 2g, Carbs: 2g.

Tarragon Air-Fried Salmon Patties

- P.T.: 25 mins
- Ingr.: 1 lb canned salmon (drained), 1 egg, ¼ cup breadcrumbs, 1 tsp tarragon, salt, pepper, olive oil spray.
- Process: Mix salmon, egg, breadcrumbs, tarragon, salt, pepper. Form patties. Spray with oil. Air fry at 370°F for 20 mins.

- Shopping list: Canned salmon, egg, breadcrumbs, tarragon, olive oil spray.
- N.I.: Calories: 180, Protein: 22g, Fat: 8g, Carbs: 6g.

Sweet and Sour Air-Fried Shrimp

- P.T.: 20 mins
- Ingr.: 1 lb shrimp, 2 tbsp sweet and sour sauce, salt, pepper, olive oil spray.
- Process: Toss shrimp in sauce, salt, pepper. Spray with oil. Air fry at 370°F for 15 mins.

- Shopping list: Shrimp, sweet and sour sauce, olive oil spray.
- N.I.: Calories: 170, Protein: 24g, Fat: 4g, Carbs: 10g.

Desserts & Sweets

Air-Fried Cinnamon Apples

- P.T.: 15 mins
- Ingr.: 2 apples (sliced), 1 tsp cinnamon, 1 tbsp honey, olive oil spray.
- Process: Toss apple slices with cinnamon and honey. Spray with oil. Air fry at 350°F for 10 mins.

- Shopping list: Apples, cinnamon, honey, olive oil spray.
- N.I.: Calories: 110, Protein: 0g, Fat: 1g, Carbs: 28g.

Banana Nut Soft Bake

- P.T.: 20 mins
- Ingr.: 2 bananas (mashed), ¼ cup walnuts (chopped), 1 tsp vanilla extract, 1 tbsp almond flour, cinnamon.
- Process: Mix bananas with walnuts, vanilla, flour, and a sprinkle of cinnamon. Air fry at 350°F for 15 mins.

- Shopping list: Bananas, walnuts, vanilla extract, almond flour.
- N.I.: Calories: 150, Protein: 3g, Fat: 8g, Carbs: 20g.

Air-Fried Peach Crumble

- P.T.: 25 mins
- Ingr.: 2 peaches (sliced), ¼ cup oats, 1 tbsp almond flour, 1 tbsp honey, ½ tsp cinnamon, olive oil spray.
- Process: Layer peach slices in a dish. Top with mixed oats, flour, honey, cinnamon. Spray with oil. Air fry at 360°F for 20 mins.
- Shopping list: Peaches, oats, almond flour, honey, cinnamon, olive oil spray.
- N.I.: Calories: 140, Protein: 3g, Fat: 3g, Carbs: 28g.

Soft Baked Pear with Honey

- P.T.: 20 mins
- Ingr.: 2 pears (halved), 2 tbsp honey, 1 tsp cinnamon, olive oil spray.
- Process: Place pear halves in the air fryer. Drizzle with honey, sprinkle cinnamon. Spray with oil. Air fry at 350°F for 15 mins.
- Shopping list: Pears, honey, cinnamon, olive oil spray.
- N.I.: Calories: 120, Protein: 1g, Fat: 1g, Carbs: 30g.

Vanilla and Berry Compote

- P.T.: 15 mins
- Ingr.: 1 cup mixed berries, 2 tbsp water, 1 tbsp sugar substitute, 1 tsp vanilla extract.
- Process: Mix berries, water, sugar substitute, vanilla in a dish. Air fry at 320°F for 10 mins.
- Shopping list: Mixed berries, sugar substitute, vanilla extract.
- N.I.: Calories: 60, Protein: 1g, Fat: 0g, Carbs: 14g.

Chocolate Avocado Pudding

- P.T.: 10 mins
- Ingr.: 1 ripe avocado, 2 tbsp cocoa powder, 1 tbsp honey, 1 tsp vanilla extract.
- Process: Blend avocado, cocoa powder, honey, vanilla until smooth.
- Shopping list: Avocado, cocoa powder, honey, vanilla extract.
- N.I.: Calories: 200, Protein: 3g, Fat: 15g, Carbs: 20g.

Air-Fried Mango Slices

- P.T.: 15 mins
- Ingr.: 1 mango (sliced), 1 tsp lime juice, a pinch of chili powder, olive oil spray.
- Process: Toss mango slices with lime juice, chili powder. Spray with oil. Air fry at 350°F for 10 mins.
- Shopping list: Mango, lime juice, chili powder, olive oil spray.
- N.I.: Calories: 100, Protein: 1g, Fat: 1g, Carbs: 25g.

Cinnamon Ricotta Cream

- P.T.: 10 mins
- Ingr.: 1 cup ricotta cheese, 1 tbsp honey, ½ tsp cinnamon.
- Process: Mix ricotta with honey and cinnamon until smooth.
- Shopping list: Ricotta cheese, honey, cinnamon.
- N.I.: Calories: 180, Protein: 10g, Fat: 10g, Carbs: 15g.

Air-Fried Stuffed Apples

- P.T.: 25 mins
- Ingr.: 2 apples (cored), 2 tbsp raisins, 1 tsp cinnamon, 1 tbsp nuts (chopped), olive oil spray.
- Process: Stuff apples with raisins, cinnamon, nuts. Spray with oil. Air fry at 340°F for 20 mins.
- Shopping list: Apples, raisins, cinnamon, nuts, olive oil spray.
- N.I.: Calories: 150, Protein: 2g, Fat: 4g, Carbs: 28g.

Soft Berry Sorbet

- P.T.: 1 hr (including freezing time)
- Ingr.: 2 cups mixed berries (frozen), 1 tbsp lemon juice, 2 tbsp water, 1 tbsp sugar substitute.
- Process: Blend berries, lemon juice, water, sugar substitute until smooth. Freeze for 1 hour.
- Shopping list: Mixed berries, lemon juice, sugar substitute.
- N.I.: Calories: 50, Protein: 1g, Fat: 0g, Carbs: 12g.

Chapter 5: Special Dietary Considerations

Recipes for Lactose Intolerance

The recipes cover various phases of the gastric sleeve bariatric diet.

Phase 1 | Almond Milk and Berry Smoothie

- P.T.: 5 mins
- Ingr.: 1 cup almond milk, ½ cup mixed berries (frozen), 1 tbsp honey.
- Process: Blend all ingredients until smooth.

- Shopping list: Almond milk, mixed berries, honey.
- N.I.: Calories: 120, Protein: 2g, Fat: 3g, Carbs: 22g.

Phase 2 | Creamy Pumpkin Soup

- P.T.: 30 mins
- Ingr.: 2 cups pumpkin puree, 1 onion (diced), 2 cups vegetable broth, 1 tsp cinnamon, salt, pepper.
- Process: Sauté onion, add pumpkin, broth, spices. Simmer and blend until smooth.

- Shopping list: Pumpkin puree, onion, vegetable broth, cinnamon.
- N.I.: Calories: 90, Protein: 2g, Fat: 1g, Carbs: 20g.

Phase 3 | Lactose-Free Chicken Parmesan

- P.T.: 30 mins
- Ingr.: 2 chicken breasts, 1 cup lactose-free mozzarella, 1 cup tomato sauce, 1 tsp Italian seasoning, olive oil, salt, pepper.
- Process: Season chicken, air fry at 360°F for 20 mins. Top with sauce, cheese. Air fry until cheese melts.
- Shopping list: Chicken breasts, lactose-free mozzarella, tomato sauce, Italian seasoning, olive oil.
- N.I.: Calories: 300, Protein: 30g, Fat: 16g, Carbs: 8g.

Phase 1 | Lactose-Free Protein Shake

- P.T.: 5 mins
- Ingr.: 1 scoop lactose-free protein powder, 1 cup almond milk, ½ banana.
- Process: Blend all ingredients until smooth.
- Shopping list: Lactose-free protein powder, almond milk, banana.
- N.I.: Calories: 180, Protein: 20g, Fat: 4g, Carbs: 20g.

Phase 2 | Mashed Cauliflower and Garlic

- P.T.: 25 mins
- Ingr.: 1 head cauliflower (chopped), 2 garlic cloves (minced), 1 tbsp olive oil, salt, pepper.
- Process: Steam cauliflower, blend with garlic, olive oil, salt, and pepper.

- Shopping list: Cauliflower, garlic, olive oil.
- N.I.: Calories: 70, Protein: 3g, Fat: 5g, Carbs: 8g.

Phase 3 | Dairy-Free Beef Stroganoff

- P.T.: 40 mins
- Ingr.: 1 lb beef strips, 1 onion (sliced), 2 cups mushrooms (sliced), 1 cup lactose-free sour cream, 1 tbsp Dijon mustard, salt, pepper, olive oil.
- Process: Sauté beef, onion, mushrooms. Add sour cream, mustard, seasonings. Simmer until creamy.

- Shopping list: Beef, onion, mushrooms, lactose-free sour cream, Dijon mustard, olive oil.
- N.I.: Calories: 300, Protein: 25g, Fat: 20g, Carbs: 10g.

Phase 1 | Lactose-Free Berry Yogurt Smoothie

- P.T.: 5 mins
- Ingr.: 1 cup lactose-free yogurt, ½ cup mixed berries (frozen), 1 tbsp honey.
- Process: Blend yogurt, berries, and honey until smooth.

- Shopping list: Lactose-free yogurt, mixed berries, honey.
- N.I.: Calories: 150, Protein: 6g, Fat: 2g, Carbs: 28g.

Phase 2 | Dairy-Free Avocado Cream Soup

- P.T.: 20 mins
- Ingr.: 2 ripe avocados, 2 cups vegetable broth, 1 lime (juiced), 1 garlic clove, salt, pepper.
- Process: Blend avocados, broth, lime juice, garlic. Heat gently.

- Shopping list: Avocados, vegetable broth, lime, garlic.
- N.I.: Calories: 200, Protein: 4g, Fat: 18g, Carbs: 12g.

Phase 3 | Lactose-Free Thai Curry Chicken

- P.T.: 30 mins
- Ingr.: 2 chicken breasts (cubed), 1 can coconut milk, 2 tbsp Thai curry paste, 1 cup mixed vegetables, 1 tsp fish sauce, salt, pepper.
- Process: Sauté chicken, add vegetables, coconut milk, curry paste, fish sauce, seasonings. Simmer until cooked.
- Shopping list: Chicken breasts, coconut milk, Thai curry paste, mixed vegetables, fish sauce.
- N.I.: Calories: 350, Protein: 25g, Fat: 25g, Carbs: 10g.

Phase 1 | Lactose-Free Creamy Carrot Ginger Juice

- P.T.: 10 mins
- Ingr.: 4 carrots, 1-inch ginger, 1 cup water, 1 tbsp almond butter.
- Process: Juice carrots, ginger. Blend with water, almond butter.
- Shopping list: Carrots, ginger, almond butter.
- N.I.: Calories: 120, Protein: 3g, Fat: 7g, Carbs: 15g.

Gluten-Free and Low-Sugar Options

The recipes cover various phases of the gastric sleeve bariatric diet.

Phase 1 | Quinoa Breakfast Bowl

- P.T.: 15 mins
- Ingr.: 1/2 cup cooked quinoa, 1/4 cup almond milk, 1/4 cup mixed berries, 1 tbsp chia seeds, 1 tsp honey.
- Process: Mix cooked quinoa with almond milk, top with berries, chia seeds, and honey.
- Shopping list: Quinoa, almond milk, mixed berries, chia seeds, honey.
- N.I.: Calories: 220, Protein: 5g, Fat: 4g, Carbs: 40g.

Phase 2 | Gluten-Free Veggie Omelette

- P.T.: 20 mins
- Ingr.: 2 eggs, 1/4 cup diced bell peppers, 1/4 cup diced tomatoes, 1/4 cup spinach leaves, salt, pepper, olive oil.
- Process: Whisk eggs, pour into a hot skillet, add veggies, cook until set.
- Shopping list: Eggs, bell peppers, tomatoes, spinach leaves, olive oil.
- N.I.: Calories: 180, Protein: 12g, Fat: 12g, Carbs: 8g.

Phase 3 | Low-Sugar Teriyaki Salmon

- P.T.: 25 mins
- Ingr.: 2 salmon fillets, 2 tbsp low-sodium teriyaki sauce, 1 tsp sesame seeds, 1 cup broccoli florets, olive oil, salt, pepper.
- Process: Brush salmon with teriyaki sauce, sprinkle sesame seeds. Air fry at 360°F for 15 mins. Steam broccoli separately.
- Shopping list: Salmon fillets, low-sodium teriyaki sauce, sesame seeds, broccoli, olive oil.
- N.I.: Calories: 320, Protein: 30g, Fat: 16g, Carbs: 10g.

Phase 1 | Almond Butter Banana Smoothie

- P.T.: 5 mins
- Ingr.: 1 cup almond milk, 1 ripe banana, 1 tbsp almond butter, 1/2 tsp cinnamon.
- Process: Blend almond milk, banana, almond butter, and cinnamon until smooth.
- Shopping list: Almond milk, ripe banana, almond butter, cinnamon.
- N.I.: Calories: 250, Protein: 4g, Fat: 11g, Carbs: 36g.

Phase 2 | Quinoa Stuffed Bell Peppers

- P.T.: 40 mins
- Ingr.: 2 bell peppers, 1/2 cup cooked quinoa, 1/4 cup black beans, 1/4 cup corn kernels, 1/4 cup diced tomatoes, 1/4 cup shredded cheddar cheese, olive oil, salt, pepper.
- Process: Hollow peppers, mix quinoa, beans, corn, tomatoes, cheese, stuff peppers. Bake at 350°F for 25 mins.
- Shopping list: Bell peppers, quinoa, black beans, corn kernels, diced tomatoes, cheddar cheese, olive oil.
- N.I.: Calories: 290, Protein: 9g, Fat: 9g, Carbs: 44g.

Phase 3 | Low-Sugar Berry Parfait

- P.T.: 10 mins
- Ingr.: 1/2 cup Greek yogurt, 1/4 cup mixed berries, 1 tbsp chopped nuts, 1 tsp honey.
- Process: Layer yogurt, berries, nuts, and honey in a glass.
- Shopping list: Greek yogurt, mixed berries, nuts, honey.
- N.I.: Calories: 180, Protein: 10g, Fat: 6g, Carbs: 20g.

Phase 1 | Gluten-Free Pancakes

- P.T.: 20 mins
- Ingr.: 1/2 cup gluten-free flour, 1/2 cup almond milk, 1 egg, 1 tbsp honey, 1/2 tsp baking powder.
- Process: Mix flour, almond milk, egg, honey, baking powder. Cook pancakes.
- Shopping list: Gluten-free flour, almond milk, egg, honey, baking powder.
- N.I.: Calories: 260, Protein: 7g, Fat: 5g, Carbs: 47g.

Phase 2 | Gluten-Free Spinach and Feta Omelette

- P.T.: 20 mins
- Ingr.: 2 eggs, 1/2 cup fresh spinach leaves, 1/4 cup crumbled feta cheese, salt, pepper, olive oil.
- Process: Whisk eggs, pour into a hot skillet, add spinach, feta, cook until set.
- Shopping list: Eggs, fresh spinach leaves, feta cheese, olive oil.
- N.I.: Calories: 230, Protein: 15g, Fat: 16g, Carbs: 4g.

Phase 3 | Low-Sugar Grilled Pineapple

- P.T.: 15 mins
- Ingr.: 4 pineapple slices, 1 tbsp honey, 1/2 tsp cinnamon.
- Process: Brush pineapple with honey, sprinkle cinnamon. Grill until caramelized.
- Shopping list: Pineapple slices, honey, cinnamon.
- N.I.: Calories: 90, Protein: 1g, Fat: 0g, Carbs: 24g.

Phase 1 | Gluten-Free Banana Muffins

- P.T.: 25 mins
- Ingr.: 2 ripe bananas, 1 cup almond flour, 1/4 cup honey, 1/2 tsp baking soda, 1/2 tsp cinnamon.
- Process: Mash bananas, mix with almond flour, honey, baking soda, and cinnamon. Bake as muffins.
- Shopping list: Ripe bananas, almond flour, honey, baking soda, cinnamon.
- N.I.: Calories: 110, Protein: 2g, Fat: 5g, Carbs: 16g.

Chapter 6: 90-Day Meal Planner

10-Day Meal Plan: Phase 1 - Liquid Diet

Day	Breakfast	Lunch	Dinner	Snack
1	Golden Turmeric Bone Broth	Healing Ginger Chicken Broth	Soothing Lemongrass Beef Broth	Citrus-Infused Fish Broth
2	Mint and Lamb Healing Broth	Spicy Tomato and Bone Broth	Herbal Turkey Broth	Asian-Style Pork Broth
3	Rosemary and Veal Bone Broth	Zingy Pepper and Chicken Broth	Cilantro Lime Seafood Broth	Earthy Mushroom and Garlic Broth
4	Soothing Carrot and Ginger Broth	Invigorating Peppermint and Lamb Broth	Ginger Infused Chicken Broth	Antioxidant Berry Blast Smoothie
5	Green Detox Juice	Tropical Mango Smoothie	Soothing Almond Milk and Vanilla Shake	Red Beet and Berry Juice
6	Carrot and Ginger Zinger Juice	Creamy Avocado and Spinach Smoothie	Blueberry Oatmeal Breakfast Smoothie	Refreshing Cucumber and Lime Juice
7	Pineapple and Ginger Immune Booster	Protein-Packed Chocolate Almond Shake	Vibrant Veggie Green Juice	Golden Milk Turmeric Smoothie
8	Spiced Apple Cinnamon Juice	Strawberry Kiwi Hydration Smoothie	Clear Vegetable Broth (If available from the recipes provided)	Almond Milk and Berry Smoothie
9	Lactose-Free Berry Yogurt Smoothie	Clear Chicken Broth (If available)	Lactose-Free Creamy Carrot Ginger Juice	Sugar-free Iced Tea (If available)
10	Almond Butter Banana Smoothie	Clear Beef Broth (If available)	Sugar-free Gelatin (If available)	Non-caffeinated Herbal Tea (If available)

10-Day Meal Plan: Phase 1 - Liquid Diet (Days 11-20)

Day	Breakfast	Lunch	Dinner	Snack
11	Herbal Turkey Broth	Asian-Style Pork Broth	Rosemary and Veal Bone Broth	Zingy Pepper and Chicken Broth
12	Cilantro Lime Seafood Broth	Earthy Mushroom and Garlic Broth	Soothing Carrot and Ginger Broth	Invigorating Peppermint and Lamb Broth
13	Ginger Infused Chicken Broth	Antioxidant Berry Blast Smoothie	Green Detox Juice	Tropical Mango Smoothie
14	Soothing Almond Milk and Vanilla Shake	Red Beet and Berry Juice	Carrot and Ginger Zinger Juice	Creamy Avocado and Spinach Smoothie
15	Blueberry Oatmeal Breakfast Smoothie	Refreshing Cucumber and Lime Juice	Pineapple and Ginger Immune Booster	Protein-Packed Chocolate Almond Shake
16	Vibrant Veggie Green Juice	Golden Milk Turmeric Smoothie	Spiced Apple Cinnamon Juice	Strawberry Kiwi Hydration Smoothie
17	Almond Milk and Berry Smoothie	Lactose-Free Creamy Carrot Ginger Juice	Lactose-Free Berry Yogurt Smoothie	Lactose-Free Protein Shake
18	Almond Butter Banana Smoothie	Citrus-Infused Fish Broth	Mint and Lamb Healing Broth	Healing Ginger Chicken Broth
19	Spicy Tomato and Bone Broth	Soothing Lemongrass Beef Broth	Golden Turmeric Bone Broth	Pineapple and Ginger Immune Booster
20	Red Beet and Berry Juice	Soothing Almond Milk and Vanilla Shake	Blueberry Oatmeal Breakfast Smoothie	Creamy Avocado and Spinach Smoothie

10-Day Meal Plan: Phase 1 - Liquid Diet (Days 21-30)

Day	Breakfast	Lunch	Dinner	Snack
21	Golden Turmeric Bone Broth	Healing Ginger Chicken Broth	Soothing Lemongrass Beef Broth	Citrus-Infused Fish Broth
22	Mint and Lamb Healing Broth	Spicy Tomato and Bone Broth	Herbal Turkey Broth	Asian-Style Pork Broth
23	Rosemary and Veal Bone Broth	Zingy Pepper and Chicken Broth	Cilantro Lime Seafood Broth	Earthy Mushroom and Garlic Broth
24	Soothing Carrot and Ginger Broth	Invigorating Peppermint Lamb Broth	Ginger Infused Chicken Broth	Antioxidant Berry Blast Smoothie
25	Green Detox Juice	Tropical Mango Smoothie	Soothing Almond Milk Vanilla Shake	Red Beet and Berry Juice
26	Carrot and Ginger Zinger Juice	Creamy Avocado and Spinach Smoothie	Blueberry Oatmeal Breakfast Smoothie	Refreshing Cucumber and Lime Juice
27	Pineapple and Ginger Immune Booster	Protein-Packed Chocolate Almond Shake	Vibrant Veggie Green Juice	Golden Milk Turmeric Smoothie
28	Spiced Apple Cinnamon Juice	Strawberry Kiwi Hydration Smoothie	Creamy Broccoli and Avocado Blend	Roasted Carrot and Ginger Puree
29	Pumpkin and White Bean Mousse	Smooth Zucchini and Basil Blend	Velvety Beet and Yogurt Puree	Cauliflower and Chive Cream
30	Sweet Potato and Cinnamon Mash	Savory Lentil and Carrot Cream	Pea and Mint Puree	Roasted Red Pepper and Walnut Spread

10-Day Meal Plan: Phase 2 - Pureed and Soft Foods (Days 31-40)

Day	Breakfast	Lunch	Dinner	Snack
31	Apple Cinnamon Oatmeal Puree	Berry Yogurt Bliss	Creamy Avocado and Banana Smoothie	Peaches and Cream Oatmeal
32	Silken Tofu and Berry Pudding	Mango Coconut Rice Pudding	Pumpkin Spice Smoothie	Almond Butter and Jelly Oatmeal
33	Cinnamon Apple Quinoa Porridge	Sweet Potato and Maple Mash	Carrot and Coriander Soup	Creamy Avocado Dip
34	Mashed Pea and Mint Spread	Roasted Red Pepper Hummus	Baked Apple and Cinnamon Puree	Sweet Potato and Ginger Soup
35	Pumpkin and Nutmeg Mousse	Creamy Beet and Feta Dip	Zucchini and Basil Velouté	Cauliflower and Parmesan Cream
36	Roasted Carrot and Ginger Puree	Creamy Broccoli and Avocado Blend	Pumpkin and White Bean Mousse	Smooth Zucchini and Basil Blend
37	Velvety Beet and Yogurt Puree	Cauliflower and Chive Cream	Sweet Potato and Cinnamon Mash	Savory Lentil and Carrot Cream
38	Pea and Mint Puree	Roasted Red Pepper and Walnut Spread	Apple Cinnamon Oatmeal Puree	Berry Yogurt Bliss
39	Creamy Avocado and Banana Smoothie	Peaches and Cream Oatmeal	Silken Tofu and Berry Pudding	Mango Coconut Rice Pudding
40	Pumpkin Spice Smoothie	Almond Butter and Jelly Oatmeal	Cinnamon Apple Quinoa Porridge	Sweet Potato and Maple Mash

10-Day Meal Plan: Phase 2 - Pureed and Soft Foods (Days 41-50)

Day	Breakfast	Lunch	Dinner	Snack
41	Berry Yogurt Bliss	Creamy Avocado and Banana Smoothie	Peaches and Cream Oatmeal	Silken Tofu and Berry Pudding
42	Mango Coconut Rice Pudding	Pumpkin Spice Smoothie	Almond Butter and Jelly Oatmeal	Cinnamon Apple Quinoa Porridge
43	Sweet Potato and Maple Mash	Carrot and Coriander Soup	Creamy Avocado Dip	Mashed Pea and Mint Spread
44	Roasted Red Pepper Hummus	Baked Apple and Cinnamon Puree	Sweet Potato and Ginger Soup	Pumpkin and Nutmeg Mousse
45	Creamy Beet and Feta Dip	Zucchini and Basil Velouté	Cauliflower and Parmesan Cream	Roasted Carrot and Ginger Puree
46	Creamy Broccoli and Avocado Blend	Pumpkin and White Bean Mousse	Smooth Zucchini and Basil Blend	Velvety Beet and Yogurt Puree
47	Cauliflower and Chive Cream	Sweet Potato and Cinnamon Mash	Savory Lentil and Carrot Cream	Pea and Mint Puree
48	Roasted Red Pepper and Walnut Spread	Apple Cinnamon Oatmeal Puree	Berry Yogurt Bliss	Creamy Avocado and Banana Smoothie
49	Peaches and Cream Oatmeal	Silken Tofu and Berry Pudding	Mango Coconut Rice Pudding	Pumpkin Spice Smoothie
50	Almond Butter and Jelly Oatmeal	Cinnamon Apple Quinoa Porridge	Sweet Potato and Maple Mash	Carrot and Coriander Soup

10-Day Meal Plan: Phase 3 - Transition to Solid Foods (Days 51-60)

Day	Breakfast	Lunch	Dinner	Snack
51	Herb-Infused Chicken Breast	Lemon Garlic Turkey Tenderloin	Spiced Ground Chicken Patties	Rosemary and Thyme Turkey Meatballs
52	Tender BBQ Chicken Thighs	Garlic Herb Roasted Turkey Breast	Balsamic Glazed Chicken Drumsticks	Simple Lemon Pepper Chicken Wings
53	Soy Glazed Turkey Meatloaf	Honey Mustard Chicken Tenders	Lemon Herb Air-Fried Salmon	Garlic Butter Air-Fried Shrimp
54	Crispy Air-Fried Tilapia	Spiced Cod Air-Fryer Delight	Herbed Shrimp and Asparagus	Air-Fried Flounder with Lemon Pepper
55	Simple Air-Fried Scallops	Lime Cilantro Air-Fried Haddock	Tarragon Air-Fried Salmon Patties	Sweet and Sour Air-Fried Shrimp
56	Air-Fried Cinnamon Apples	Banana Nut Soft Bake	Air-Fried Peach Crumble	Soft Baked Pear with Honey
57	Vanilla and Berry Compote	Chocolate Avocado Pudding	Air-Fried Mango Slices	Cinnamon Ricotta Cream
58	Air-Fried Stuffed Apples	Soft Berry Sorbet	Almond Milk and Berry Smoothie	Creamy Pumpkin Soup
59	Lactose-Free Chicken Parmesan	Lactose-Free Protein Shake	Mashed Cauliflower and Garlic	Dairy-Free Beef Stroganoff
60	Lactose-Free Berry Yogurt Smoothie	Dairy-Free Avocado Cream Soup	Lactose-Free Thai Curry Chicken	Lactose-Free Creamy Carrot Ginger Juice

10-Day Meal Plan: Phase 3 - Transition to Solid Foods (Days 61-70)

Day	Breakfast	Lunch	Dinner	Snack
61	Lemon Herb Air-Fried Salmon	Garlic Butter Air-Fried Shrimp	Crispy Air-Fried Tilapia	Spiced Cod Air-Fryer Delight
62	Herbed Shrimp and Asparagus	Air-Fried Flounder with Lemon Pepper	Simple Air-Fried Scallops	Lime Cilantro Air-Fried Haddock
63	Tarragon Air-Fried Salmon Patties	Sweet and Sour Air-Fried Shrimp	Air-Fried Cinnamon Apples	Banana Nut Soft Bake
64	Air-Fried Peach Crumble	Soft Baked Pear with Honey	Vanilla and Berry Compote	Chocolate Avocado Pudding
65	Air-Fried Mango Slices	Cinnamon Ricotta Cream	Air-Fried Stuffed Apples	Soft Berry Sorbet
66	Quinoa Breakfast Bowl	Gluten-Free Veggie Omelette	Low-Sugar Teriyaki Salmon	Almond Butter Banana Smoothie
67	Quinoa Stuffed Bell Peppers	Low-Sugar Berry Parfait	Gluten-Free Pancakes	Gluten-Free Spinach and Feta Omelette
68	Low-Sugar Grilled Pineapple	Gluten-Free Banana Muffins	Herb-Infused Chicken Breast	Lemon Garlic Turkey Tenderloin
69	Spiced Ground Chicken Patties	Rosemary and Thyme Turkey Meatballs	Tender BBQ Chicken Thighs	Garlic Herb Roasted Turkey Breast
70	Balsamic Glazed Chicken Drumsticks	Simple Lemon Pepper Chicken Wings	Soy Glazed Turkey Meatloaf	Honey Mustard Chicken Tenders

10-Day Meal Plan: Phase 3 - Transition to Solid Foods (Days 71-80)

Day	Breakfast	Lunch	Dinner	Snack
71	Gluten-Free Banana Muffins	Low-Sugar Grilled Pineapple	Herb-Infused Chicken Breast	Lemon Garlic Turkey Tenderloin
72	Spiced Ground Chicken Patties	Rosemary and Thyme Turkey Meatballs	Tender BBQ Chicken Thighs	Garlic Herb Roasted Turkey Breast
73	Balsamic Glazed Chicken Drumsticks	Simple Lemon Pepper Chicken Wings	Soy Glazed Turkey Meatloaf	Honey Mustard Chicken Tenders
74	Lemon Herb Air-Fried Salmon	Garlic Butter Air-Fried Shrimp	Crispy Air-Fried Tilapia	Spiced Cod Air-Fryer Delight
75	Herbed Shrimp and Asparagus	Air-Fried Flounder with Lemon Pepper	Simple Air-Fried Scallops	Lime Cilantro Air-Fried Haddock
76	Tarragon Air-Fried Salmon Patties	Sweet and Sour Air-Fried Shrimp	Air-Fried Cinnamon Apples	Banana Nut Soft Bake
77	Air-Fried Peach Crumble	Soft Baked Pear with Honey	Vanilla and Berry Compote	Chocolate Avocado Pudding
78	Air-Fried Mango Slices	Cinnamon Ricotta Cream	Air-Fried Stuffed Apples	Soft Berry Sorbet
79	Quinoa Breakfast Bowl	Gluten-Free Veggie Omelette	Low-Sugar Teriyaki Salmon	Almond Butter Banana Smoothie
80	Quinoa Stuffed Bell Peppers	Low-Sugar Berry Parfait	Gluten-Free Pancakes	Gluten-Free Spinach and Feta Omelette

10-Day Meal Plan: Phase 3 - Transition to Solid Foods (Days 81-90)

Day	Breakfast	Lunch	Dinner	Snack
81	Lemon Herb Air-Fried Salmon	Garlic Butter Air-Fried Shrimp	Crispy Air-Fried Tilapia	Spiced Cod Air-Fryer Delight
82	Herbed Shrimp and Asparagus	Air-Fried Flounder with Lemon Pepper	Simple Air-Fried Scallops	Lime Cilantro Air-Fried Haddock
83	Tarragon Air-Fried Salmon Patties	Sweet and Sour Air-Fried Shrimp	Air-Fried Cinnamon Apples	Banana Nut Soft Bake
84	Air-Fried Peach Crumble	Soft Baked Pear with Honey	Vanilla and Berry Compote	Chocolate Avocado Pudding
85	Air-Fried Mango Slices	Cinnamon Ricotta Cream	Air-Fried Stuffed Apples	Soft Berry Sorbet
86	Lemon Garlic Turkey Tenderloin	Spiced Ground Chicken Patties	Rosemary and Thyme Turkey Meatballs	Tender BBQ Chicken Thighs
87	Garlic Herb Roasted Turkey Breast	Balsamic Glazed Chicken Drumsticks	Simple Lemon Pepper Chicken Wings	Soy Glazed Turkey Meatloaf
88	Honey Mustard Chicken Tenders	Lemon Herb Air-Fried Salmon	Garlic Butter Air-Fried Shrimp	Crispy Air-Fried Tilapia
89	Spiced Cod Air-Fryer Delight	Herbed Shrimp and Asparagus	Air-Fried Flounder with Lemon Pepper	Simple Air-Fried Scallops
90	Lime Cilantro Air-Fried Haddock	Tarragon Air-Fried Salmon Patties	Sweet and Sour Air-Fried Shrimp	Air-Fried Cinnamon Apples

Chapter 7: Maintenance and Moving Forward

Staying on Track: The Art of Long-Term Success

When embarking on a journey to better health through the gastric sleeve bariatric diet, you are not merely seeking a short-term solution but a lasting transformation. Staying on track is the linchpin to achieving and maintaining the positive changes you've worked so hard for. In this section, we will explore the art of long-term success, sharing insights, strategies, and anecdotes to help you remain steadfast on your path.

The Bariatric Odyssey: A Lifelong Commitment

The decision to undergo gastric sleeve surgery and embrace a bariatric lifestyle is a profound one, often born out of a desire for better health and an improved quality of life. As you embark on this journey, it's important to recognize that it's not a one-time event but a lifelong commitment. Your body, your relationship with food, and your perspective on health will undergo significant transformations, but they require continuous nurturing and care.

The Importance of Staying on Track

Why is staying on track so crucial? It's because long-term success in bariatric surgery isn't solely about the number on the scale; it's about the holistic well-being of your body and mind. Here's why it matters:

1. Health Benefits: The primary goal of gastric sleeve surgery is to improve your health. Staying on track with your dietary and lifestyle changes ensures that you continue to reap the benefits, such as better blood sugar control, reduced risk of heart disease, and improved mobility.

2. Sustained Weight Loss: Maintaining a healthy weight is a key objective. Staying on track with your dietary guidelines helps you achieve and sustain your target weight, preventing the regaining of lost pounds.

3. Emotional Well-Being: Achieving and maintaining your desired weight is often accompanied by improved self-esteem and a more positive body image. Staying on track nurtures your emotional well-being, fostering a healthier relationship with yourself.

4. Nutritional Sufficiency: The gastric sleeve bariatric diet is designed to provide essential nutrients while restricting caloric intake. Staying on track ensures that you receive the nutrition your body needs for optimal functioning.

5. Longevity: A commitment to staying on track translates into a longer and healthier life. It reduces the risk of obesity-related comorbidities and enhances your overall longevity.

Strategies for Staying on Track

Now that we've established the significance of staying on track, let's explore practical strategies to help you maintain your focus and determination:

1. Personalized Meal Planning: Your bariatric journey is unique to you. Work with a registered dietitian to create a personalized meal plan that aligns with your dietary phase, preferences, and nutritional needs. Having a tailored plan makes it easier to stay on track.

2. Mindful Eating: Cultivate mindfulness in your eating habits. Pay attention to hunger and fullness cues, savor each bite, and avoid distractions during meals. Mindful eating fosters a healthier relationship with food.

3. Regular Exercise: Incorporating regular physical activity into your routine is vital. Consult with your healthcare provider to determine the appropriate level of exercise based on your progress. Exercise not only supports weight maintenance but also enhances overall well-being.

4. Support System: Lean on your support system. Whether it's friends, family, or a support group, sharing your journey and challenges with others can provide valuable encouragement and accountability.

5. Hydration: Proper hydration is essential. Aim to drink enough water throughout the day. Staying hydrated supports digestion and helps prevent overeating.

6. Portion Control: Continue to be mindful of portion sizes, even as you transition to solid foods. Use smaller plates and utensils to help control your portions effectively.

7. Regular Check-Ups: Don't skip follow-up appointments with your healthcare team. These check-ups are crucial for monitoring your progress and making necessary adjustments to your diet and lifestyle.

8. Celebrate Achievements: Acknowledge and celebrate your achievements along the way. Whether it's reaching a weight milestone, trying a new healthy recipe, or completing a fitness challenge, celebrating these successes can boost your motivation.

The Challenges You May Encounter

While the gastric sleeve bariatric diet offers numerous benefits, it also presents its share of challenges. It's essential to anticipate and address these challenges to stay on track effectively.

Addressing Common Challenges: Navigating the Bumps in the Road

While the path to long-term success on the gastric sleeve bariatric diet is rewarding, it's not without its challenges. In this section, we'll explore some common roadblocks you may encounter and provide guidance on how to navigate them successfully.

1. Plateauing Progress

At some point in your journey, you might find that your weight loss progress has slowed or even come to a halt. This plateau can be frustrating, but it's a common occurrence. Here's how to address it:

Solution: Instead of solely focusing on the number on the scale, shift your attention to other indicators of progress. Track changes in your body measurements, energy levels, and overall well-being. Plateaus can also be an opportunity to reassess your dietary habits and exercise routine. Consult with your healthcare team for personalized advice.

2. Emotional Eating

Emotional eating is a challenge for many individuals, and it can resurface even after bariatric surgery. Stress, boredom, or emotional triggers can lead to overeating.

Solution: Develop alternative coping strategies for dealing with emotions. Practice mindfulness techniques, engage in hobbies you enjoy, or seek support from a therapist or support group. Building emotional resilience is key to overcoming emotional eating.

3. Food Cravings

Cravings for unhealthy foods may occasionally arise, tempting you to deviate from your dietary guidelines.

Solution: Remember the reasons you embarked on this journey. Visualize your health goals and the positive changes you've experienced. When cravings strike, distract yourself with a favorite activity or opt for healthier alternatives that align with your dietary phase.

4. Social Pressures

Social gatherings and events can pose challenges as they often revolve around food. Navigating these situations while adhering to your dietary guidelines can be tricky.

Solution: Communicate your dietary needs with friends and family. They may be more understanding and accommodating than you anticipate. You can also eat a small, nutritious meal before attending events to reduce the temptation to overindulge.

5. Feeling Isolated

Embarking on a bariatric journey can sometimes lead to feelings of isolation or the sense that you're facing the challenges alone.

Solution: Seek support from a bariatric support group or therapist. Sharing your experiences and challenges with others who have undergone similar journeys can provide valuable camaraderie and advice. You are not alone in this.

6. Digestive Issues

Gastrointestinal symptoms like dumping syndrome or food intolerances can be unsettling.

Solution: If you experience digestive issues, consult with your healthcare provider. They can help identify triggers and provide guidance on managing symptoms. It's essential to follow your dietary guidelines to minimize discomfort.

7. Regaining Weight

While maintaining weight loss is a primary goal, some individuals may experience weight regain over time.

Solution: If you find yourself regaining weight, it's essential to address it promptly. Consult with your healthcare team to evaluate your dietary and exercise habits. They can help you develop a plan to get back on track.

8. Staying Active

Incorporating regular physical activity into your routine can be challenging, especially if you have a sedentary lifestyle.

Solution: Start with small, manageable goals. Aim to increase your physical activity gradually. Find activities you enjoy, whether it's walking, swimming, or dancing. Remember that every step counts towards improving your health.

9. Maintaining Motivation

Sustaining motivation for the long haul can be tough. As time passes, the initial excitement of your journey may wane.

Solution: Revisit your health goals regularly. Celebrate your achievements, no matter how small. Consider creating a vision board or journaling about your progress. Surround yourself with positive reminders of why you started this journey.

10. Adequate Hydration
Staying hydrated is vital but can be challenging, especially if you're prone to sipping on beverages throughout the day.

Solution: Set hydration goals and use a reusable water bottle to track your intake. Experiment with different flavored water or herbal teas to make staying hydrated more enjoyable.

Addressing these common challenges requires patience, resilience, and a commitment to your well-being. Remember that setbacks are a natural part of any journey. What matters most is how you respond to them. Embrace these challenges as opportunities for growth and continue moving forward on your path to lasting health and happiness.

Celebrating Milestones and Successes: Acknowledging Your Achievements

As you progress on your journey, you'll reach significant weight loss milestones, representing your dedication and hard work paying off. Celebrate by treating yourself to non-food rewards, such as purchasing new clothing that fits your changing body or indulging in a spa day. Reflect on how far you've come and acknowledge your resilience.

Bariatric surgery often leads to improvements in various health markers, such as lower blood pressure, improved blood sugar control, and reduced cholesterol levels. Celebrate these improvements by scheduling regular check-ups with your healthcare provider. Witnessing positive changes in your health parameters can be highly motivating.

Adhering to the dietary guidelines of your specific phase is an achievement in itself. Each phase transition marks a significant step toward reclaiming your health. Share your dietary achievements with loved ones by hosting a small gathering with friends and family, preparing bariatric-friendly dishes to showcase your progress.

Gradually increasing your physical activity level is a significant accomplishment, whether it's walking a certain distance or mastering a new exercise routine. Treat yourself to fitness-related rewards, such as new workout gear or a fitness tracker. Tracking your progress and setting new fitness goals can be empowering.

Improved emotional well-being is often an overlooked success. Bariatric surgery can lead to enhanced self-confidence and a more positive self-image. Engage in self-care activities that promote emotional well-being, such as meditation, journaling, or spending quality time with loved ones who support your journey.

Being part of a supportive bariatric community is a success in itself. Connecting with others who share similar experiences can be incredibly empowering. Attend bariatric support group meetings or online forums regularly and share your experiences and knowledge with fellow community members. Your insights can inspire and motivate others.

As you transition to solid foods, exploring a wider variety of foods and flavors is an exciting achievement. Host a themed meal night where you prepare dishes from different cultures or cuisines. Experimenting with new recipes can make your dietary journey more enjoyable.

Non-scale victories encompass all the positive changes in your life that extend beyond the numbers on the scale, such as improved sleep, increased energy, and a better quality of life. Keep a journal of your non-scale victories and reflect on how these changes have positively impacted your daily life. Share your triumphs with your support network.

Taking time to express gratitude for your journey and reflect on your successes is a valuable practice. Create a gratitude journal where you jot down the things you're grateful for each day. Regularly revisit your journal to remind yourself of the progress you've made.

Once you've experienced success on your bariatric journey, consider giving back by supporting others who are starting their path to health. Volunteer your time with bariatric support groups or mentor individuals who are about to undergo surgery. Being a source of guidance and inspiration is a meaningful way to celebrate your achievements.

Conclusion & Your Next Steps: A Journey Beyond Surgery

As we conclude this comprehensive guide to the gastric sleeve bariatric diet, it's essential to acknowledge the significant transformation you've embarked on. Your decision to undergo bariatric surgery and commit to a new way of life is a testament to your determination, courage, and the profound desire for a healthier and more fulfilling future. While this guide has equipped you with the knowledge and tools to navigate the various phases of the diet, it's crucial to recognize that your journey extends far beyond the surgical suite and the immediate post-operative period.

Take a moment to reflect on how far you've come. From the initial decision to explore bariatric surgery to the preparation, the surgery itself, and the phases of the diet, your journey has been marked by significant milestones. These milestones represent not only physical changes but also a shift in your mindset and lifestyle. Acknowledge your resilience and celebrate your achievements, no matter how small they may seem.

One of the most profound changes you've experienced is your relationship with food. Bariatric surgery has altered the way your body processes and interacts with nourishment. You've learned to savor each bite, prioritize nutrient-dense foods, and listen to your body's cues. As you move forward, continue to nurture this mindful approach to eating. Remember that food is fuel for your body, and your choices should align with your health and well-being.

Physical activity has become an integral part of your life. Whether it's daily walks, structured workouts, or active hobbies, you've discovered the joy of movement. Maintain this commitment to an active lifestyle. Explore new activities, set fitness goals, and revel in the vitality that regular exercise brings. Staying active is not only essential for weight management but also for your overall health and longevity.

Your journey has also touched on emotional well-being. Bariatric surgery often leads to improved self-confidence and emotional health. Continue to prioritize self-care, both in terms of physical and emotional well-being. Practice self-compassion, engage in stress-reducing activities, and seek support when needed. Your emotional health is as crucial as your physical health on this journey.

Your support network has played a pivotal role in your success. Friends, family, healthcare providers, and fellow bariatric community members have been sources of encouragement and guidance. Stay connected with these individuals who understand your journey intimately. Share your experiences, provide support to others, and draw strength from your community.

While you've achieved remarkable success, remember that your journey is ongoing. Set new goals and aspirations. These can encompass various aspects of your life, from further weight loss and fitness achievements to career ambitions and personal growth. Continually challenging yourself and striving for improvement will keep your journey dynamic and fulfilling.

Maintain regular check-ups with your healthcare provider. These appointments are vital for monitoring your progress, addressing any potential issues, and ensuring your long-term health and well-being. It's crucial to stay vigilant and proactive in managing your health.

Consider paying it forward by inspiring and supporting others who are beginning their bariatric journey. Your experiences, insights, and successes can serve as valuable guidance for individuals taking their first steps toward a healthier life. Being a source of inspiration and mentorship is a meaningful way to contribute to the bariatric community.

As you move forward, remember that your journey is unique. Embrace the lessons you've learned and the growth you've experienced. Continue to prioritize your health, well-being, and personal development. Your path may encounter challenges, but with the resilience and determination you've demonstrated, there's no obstacle you cannot overcome.

Acknowledgments: Gratitude for Support and Inspiration

In the culmination of this comprehensive guide to the gastric sleeve bariatric diet, it is with immense gratitude and heartfelt appreciation that we acknowledge the individuals and sources that have contributed to the creation of this resource. Our journey in providing you with valuable information and guidance would not have been possible without the support, expertise, and inspiration of many.

First and foremost, we extend our deepest appreciation to the healthcare professionals and experts in the field of bariatric surgery and nutrition. Their dedication to improving the lives of individuals through surgical intervention and dietary guidance is nothing short of remarkable. We are grateful for their commitment to patient care and for sharing their expertise to empower individuals on their bariatric journeys.

To the patients and individuals who have embarked on the transformative path of bariatric surgery, we extend our heartfelt gratitude. Your stories, experiences, and resilience have served as a wellspring of inspiration. Your determination to reclaim your health and well-being is a testament to the human spirit's capacity for positive change.

We express our gratitude to the supportive families and friends of bariatric patients. Your unwavering encouragement, understanding, and patience have been instrumental in the success of your loved ones. Your role as pillars of support cannot be overstated, and we acknowledge the sacrifices you've made to uplift those on their bariatric journeys.

To the broader bariatric community, including support groups, online forums, and organizations dedicated to bariatric health, we extend our appreciation. Your platforms provide a vital network for individuals to connect, share experiences, and seek guidance. Your commitment to fostering a sense of community and belonging is commendable.

The extensive research and medical literature that have informed this guide deserve recognition. We are grateful for the wealth of knowledge contributed by researchers, clinicians, and healthcare institutions worldwide. Their dedication to advancing the understanding of bariatric surgery, nutrition, and health outcomes has paved the way for improved patient care.

Our appreciation extends to the diverse culinary traditions and the creative minds behind the recipes featured in this guide. Food is not only nourishment but also a source of joy and cultural richness. We thank the culinary experts and chefs who have shared their expertise in crafting flavorful and nutritious recipes tailored to the bariatric journey.

We acknowledge the tireless efforts of our editorial and design teams who have worked diligently to present this guide in a visually appealing and informative format. Their dedication to clarity and excellence in communication is evident in every page.

Last but not least, we express our gratitude to you, the reader. Your commitment to seeking knowledge and embracing a healthier lifestyle is at the heart of this guide's purpose. We hope that the information and insights presented here serve as a valuable resource on your journey toward improved health and well-being.

Made in the USA
Monee, IL
31 December 2024